Fundamental Biomechanics

Includes PPT with Computer Graphic for Teachers and Students

AKOUETEVI ADUAYOM-AHEGO

EHARA YOSHIHIRO

SARAH R. CHANG

GARY GUERRA

Copyright © 2021 Akouetevi Aduayom-Ahego, Ehara Yoshihiro, Sarah R. Chang, Gary Guerra.

All rights reserved. No part of this book may be reproduced, stored, or transmitted by any means—whether auditory, graphic, mechanical, or electronic—without written permission of both publisher and author, except in the case of brief excerpts used in critical articles and reviews. Unauthorized reproduction of any part of this work is illegal and is punishable by law.

Cover Design by 100Covers.com
Interior Design by FormattedBooks.com

Original Authors

Yamamoto Sumiko	International University of Health and Welfare
IIshii Shinichirou	International University of Health and Welfare
Ehara Yoshihiro	Niigata University of Health and Welfare

This book was originally published in Japanese under the title of:
Kiso Baiomekanikusu (Fundamental Biomechanics, 2nd edition.)
© 2015 ISHIYAKU PUBLISHERS, INC.7-10, Honkomagome 1 chome, Bunkyo-ku, Tokyo 113-8612, Japan
No part of this textbook may be reproduced in any form without the permission from the publisher.

Translated by

Akouetevi Aduayom-Ahego	Dream GP Inc., Japan / University of Health and Allied Sciences, Ghana
Ehara Yoshihiro	Niigata University of Health and Welfare, Japan
Sarah R. Chang	Orthocare Innovations, USA
Gary Guerra	Mahidol University, Thailand

Copyright © 2021, Akouetevi Aduayom-Ahego, Ehara Yoshihiro.
All rights reserved. No part of this textbook may be reproduced in any form without the permission from the authors.

2022 January

About the translating authors

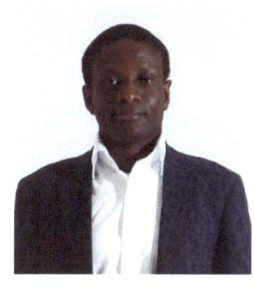

Akouetevi Aduayom-Ahego, Ph.D. is a faculty member in the Department of Orthotics and Prosthetics, School of Allied Health Sciences, University of Health and Allied Sciences, Ghana. He studied Prosthetics & Orthotics at Ecole Nationale des Auxiliaires Médicaux, Togo. He completed his both Msc in Rehabilitation and Ph.D. in Health Science at Niigata University of Health and Welfare, Japan. He worked as Research Associate in the Faculty of Sport Sciences at Waseda University. His research interest is in biomechanics and development of Prosthetics & Orthotics education and service in low-income countries.

Ehara Yoshihiro, Ph.D. is a Biomechanical Engineer. He teaches biomechanics to students of Physical Therapy, Occupational Therapy, Prosthetics & Orthotics at the Niigata University of Health and Welfare. He organized a lot of biomechanics seminar all over Japan and also in Thailand.

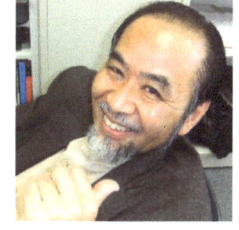

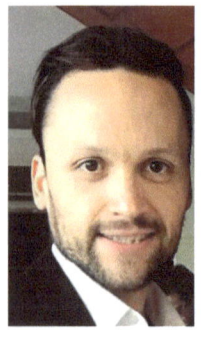 **Gary Guerra, Ph.D.** is a faculty member in the Sirindhorn School of Prosthetics and Orthotics, Faculty of Medicine, Siriraj Hospital, Mahidol University. His interests span from physical activity monitoring to exercise testing of prosthesis wearers. He received his Ph.D. from Loma Linda University in Rehabilitation Science, post-graduate certificate in Prosthetics from California State University Dominguez Hills, and master and undergraduate degrees in Kinesiology from Texas A&M University San Antonio.

Sarah R. Chang, Ph.D. is the Director of Research & Development at Orthocare Innovations, LLC focused on research and development of prosthetic, orthotic, and assistive device technologies. She received her B.S. in Biomedical Engineering from California Polytechnic State University, San Luis Obispo and Ph.D. in Biomedical Engineering from Case Western Reserve University. Her commercial and research interests use biomechanics and engineering to improve mobility in individuals with disabilities.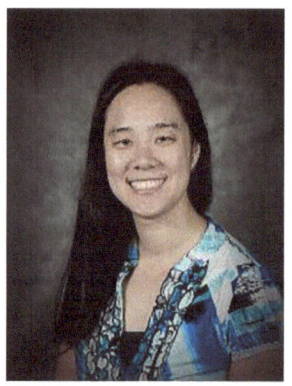

Preface of the Original Book

Professor Yamamoto and I have been conducting motion analysis seminars since 1995. For decades, we have been organizing seminars across Japan from Hokkaido to Okinawa twice a year. The seminars were scheduled for four-days, with a maximum of 30 participants. We conducted data collection, performed analyses and ended each seminar with a final presentation. Through this process, we have been able to analyze five main biomechanical parameters such as the center of gravity, ground reaction force, center of pressure, joint moment, and joint power. These seminars attracted many repeat attendees, which has led to improvements in content of seminars and value for the academic's attendees. Regular participants of these seminars have been Physical Therapists (PT), Medical Doctors, Occupational Therapists (OT), Prosthetists / Orthotists (PO), Nurses, Care Workers, Rehabilitation Engineers and Sport Science professionals. The content of these seminars has also been implemented into PT student education. As a result, separate motion analysis seminars have been routinely organized by PT students. For decades, we have been fortunate to have trained over a thousand participants.

However, this transmission of fundamental knowledge of biomechanics has yet to reach the wide spread audience of international professionals. From 2009, biomechanics seminars for faculty staff from universities and colleges have been organized. The content of these seminars primarily focused on practical training with topics such as, force synthesis and lever systems as well as motion and gait biomechanics. Though the seminars were well received, the ideal practicum of these seminars is one which allows for faculty and staff to gain fundamental knowledge whilst practicing biomechanics. This textbook was published for this purpose. As such, this book is useful for educators and students alike. The book makes an excellent textbook; as it was also edited for student self-learning. It is my hope that both educators and students can gain a thorough understanding of fundamental biomechanics.

Yoshihiro Ehara

Preface

This textbook describes the basic principles of Biomechanics. This book was originally published in the Japanese language and authored by Prof. Yamamoto Sumiko, Prof. Ishii Shinichirou and Prof. Ehara Yoshihiro. During my master and doctoral studies in Prof. Ehara's laboratory at Niigata University of Health and Welfare, I found the text very practical for both teaching faculty as well as students. The book illustrates in a detailed manner, the characteristics of forces applied to human movement. It will be useful for academics and professionals in Allied Health Sciences such as: Physical Rehabilitation, Ergonomics, Physical Therapy, Occupational Therapy, Prosthetics / Orthotics and Sport Sciences. Little attention has been paid to the practical dissemination of Applied Biomechanics instruction in resource limited environments due to the high cost of laboratory equipment. This textbook utilizes computer graphics to comprehensively explain biomechanics of human motion such as gait, squatting, sit to stand movements and more. This simplified textbook will be an asset for Universities, professionals, researchers, students and those interested in motion analysis residing in both developed and resource limited environments.

Akouetevi Aduayom-Ahego

How to use this textbook

This textbook is designed for both teachers and students. The figures in the main text are also represented in the Power Point file. Teachers are free to edit the contents of the Power Point as reference while using this textbook to teach students in their program. Some of the computer graphics in the slides can be played to show motion such as squatting, the trajectory of center of gravity and center of pressure, jumping, sit to stand, gait initiation and so on.

The Power Point file can be requested through the link below:

https://ahelitebrace.com/fundamental-biomechanics

After downloading the Power Point file, use the access passcode: **AH2020@FB**

Contents

Chapter 1 Synthesis and Decomposition of Force 1
On completion of this chapter, you will be able:
1. To explain the synthesis of forces
2. To explain the decomposition of forces
3. To explain how to synthesize and decompose forces

Chapter 2 Applications of the Lever System to the Living Body 13
On completion of this chapter, you will be able:
1. To understand the lever systems
2. To understand the application methods of the lever systems on the human body

Chapter 3 Center of Gravity (COG) calculation 27
On completion of this chapter, you will be able:
1. To explain the lever systems
2. To explain the concept of the center of gravity
3. To explain how to calculate the center of gravity
4. To understand how a change of posture affects the center of gravity

Chapter 4 Velocity and Acceleration of the Center of Gravity 37
On completion of this chapter, you will be able:
1. To explain the velocity of the center of gravity
2. To explain the acceleration of the center of gravity
3. To draw a graph of the velocity of the center of gravity when standing up and sitting down
4. To draw a graph of the acceleration of the center of gravity when standing up and sitting down

Chapter 5   Ground Reaction Force and COG Acceleration 49
On completion of this chapter, you will be able:
1. To explain the relationship between the force and the acceleration of the COG
2. To explain the ground reaction force exerted on the body
3. To explain the relationship between the ground reaction force and the movement of the COG during squatting

Chapter 6   Center of Pressure (COP) 63
On completion of this chapter, you will be able:
1. To explain the meaning of Center of Pressure
2. To explain the relationship between Center of Pressure and base of support
3. To explain the relationship between the Center of Pressure and the center of gravity position
4. To explain the character of the center of gravity, the ground reaction force and the Center of Pressure during standing, sitting and reach movements

Chapter 7   Joint Moments and Muscular Activities 75
On completion of this chapter, you will be able:
1. To explain joint moments
2. To tell how to calculate the joint moments
3. To explain the relationship between joint moments and ground reaction forces

Chapter 8   Joint Power 85
On completion of this chapter, you will be able:
1. To explain the meaning of joint power
2. To explain mechanical work
3. To explain the work generated by muscles
4. To explain the power generated by muscles
5. To explain the relationship between power and muscle contraction

Chapter 9 Jump Movement..95
On completion of this chapter, you will be able:
1. To explain mechanical energy
2. To explain muscle activity and jump height
3. To explain ground reaction force and center of gravity acceleration during jumping
4. To explain the joint moments during jumping
5. To explain the power of joint moments during jumping
6. To explain how to jump high

Chapter 10 Biomechanics while Rising from a Chair........................ 105
On completion of this chapter, you will be able:
1. To explain the movement of the center of gravity while rising from a chair
2. To explain the meaning of the trunk tilting forward
3. To explain the change in the base of support and center of pressure
4. To explain changes in ground reaction force
5. To explain the activities of muscles while rising from a chair

Chapter 11 Biomechanics of Gait Initiation....................................... 115
On completion of this chapter, you will be able:
1. To explain the relationship between the center of gravity and COP when standing upright
2. To explain the movement of COP in sagittal and frontal planes during gait initiation
3. To explain the relationship between the movement of COG and COP
4. To explain the relationship between COP movement and joint moment
5. To explain the driving force to move the COG forward

Chapter 12 Gait Biomechanics, Center of Gravity and Center of Pressure During Walking... 123
On completion of this chapter, you will be able:
1. To explain the relationship between the center of gravity and center of pressure during walking
2. To explain the relationship between the center of pressure and joint moment during walking
3. To explain the relationship between the movement of the center of gravity and the ground reaction force

**Chapter 13 Functions to Smooth the Center of Gravity
Movement During Gait** **133**
On completion of this chapter, you will be able:
1. To explain the function to smooth the movement of the center of gravity during walking
2. To explain the shock absorption mechanism during walking
3. To explain the relationship between the rocker function and the smooth movement of the center of gravity

**Chapter 14 Observational Gait Analysis OGIG method
Observational Gait Instructor Group** **141**
On completion of this chapter, you will be able:
1. To explain OGIG gait terms
2. To explain the standard joint angle of healthy subjects in each gait cycle
3. To explain the three rocker functions

CHAPTER 1

Synthesis and Decomposition of Force

On completion of this chapter, you will be able:

1. To explain the synthesis of forces
2. To explain the decomposition of forces
3. To explain how to synthesize and decompose forces

Synthesis and decomposition of forces are the most fundamental concept among biomechanics. In this chapter, you will learn the theory and the method for synthesizing and decomposing forces.

Synthesis and Decomposition of Force

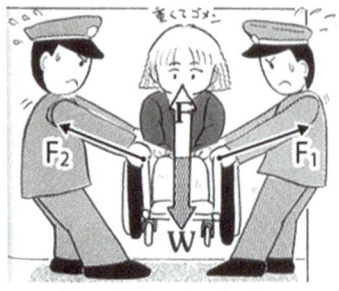

Manga Biomechanics 1, Nankodo, Tokyo, 1994

Let us consider an example of lifting up a woman in a wheelchair by two people. In this case, the force F, which is the combined forces of F1 and F2 exerted by each of the station staff, will support the gravitational force W applied to the wheelchair and her body. In this case, the synthesis of F1 and F2 becomes F. Now, think of how you can synthesize the two forces.

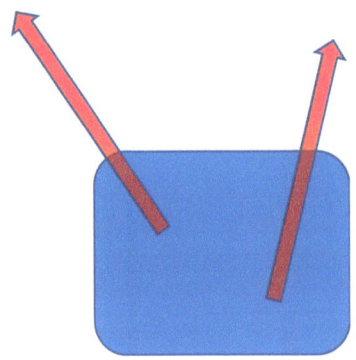

Synthesis of forces in different directions
In the example above, forces F1 and F2 were left-right symmetrically. Let's consider that the forces exerted by the two-station staff are not left-right symmetrical. This arrangement will be a more general situation of the two forces. How would you synthesize the two forces?

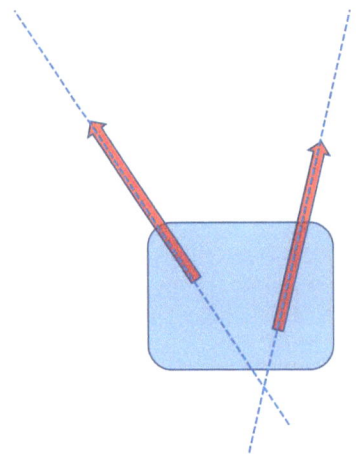

\<Hint\>
First, extend the line of action of each force.

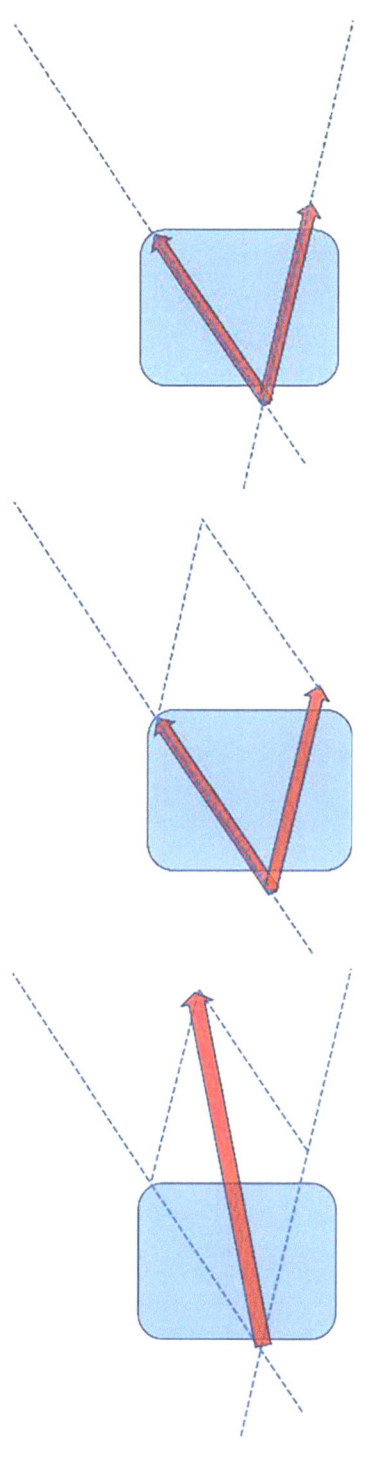

Let's consider the intersection as the origin. The two forces can be moved along their lines of action so that each base of the forces reaches the origin.

Consider the tips of the two arrows as a vertex to draw a parallelogram as shown in the figure.

Draw a diagonal line from the origin to the opposite vertex in the parallelogram which represents the resultant force.

Synthesis and Decomposition of Force

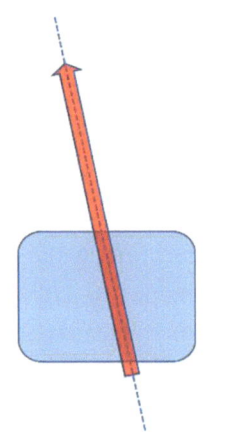

Let's consider the extension of the line of action of the resultant force. The synthesized force can be moved along the line of action. This movement does not change the action of the force. In other words, you can move a force to anywhere you think on the line of action. This is the method of synthesizing two forces in different directions. In this case, the resultant force was not exactly vertical to the horizontal line, because the two forces were not left-right symmetrical.

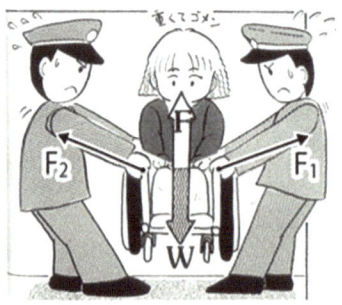

Manga Biomechanics 1, Nankodo, Tokyo, 1994

Let's go back to the example of lifting the wheelchair by the two station staffs described already. If the direction of the resultant force is not exactly vertical to the horizontal line, the wheelchair will not be raised properly and safely. To properly pull up the wheelchair directly upward, the two-station staff should have pulled left-right (horizontal) symmetrically.

In this situation, the horizontal component of F1 and F2 are canceled out by each other and cause no effect to lift the wheelchair and the woman.

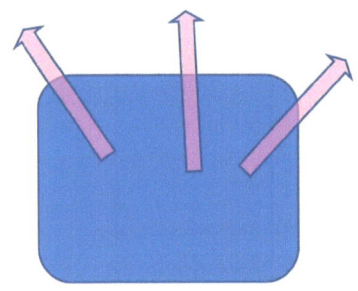

Synthesis of three or more forces

For the next application, consider the synthesis of three forces. **Question:** what is the resultant force of synthesizing these three forces? First, estimate the resultant of the left and middle two forces to make one resultant force. We will then have two forces. Finally, synthesize the remaining two forces to generate the final force. Therefore, three forces become one force. Try to answer this question by yourself.

Fundamental Biomechanics

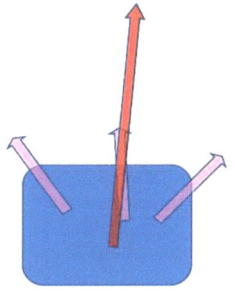

The red arrow shows the correct answer. Please verify the answer by yourself.

Synthesis of parallel forces

In the previous example, we described the synthesis of two forces of different directions.

If the two forces have the same direction, in other words, parallel, the previous method cannot be used because the line of action does not have an intersection point. In such cases, proceed as follows. First, let's consider an example where both forces have the same magnitude of 10 N.

In this case, the magnitude of the resultant force is twice the forces of each side, which is 10 N + 10 N = 20 N. The action line goes through the midpoint of the two forces.

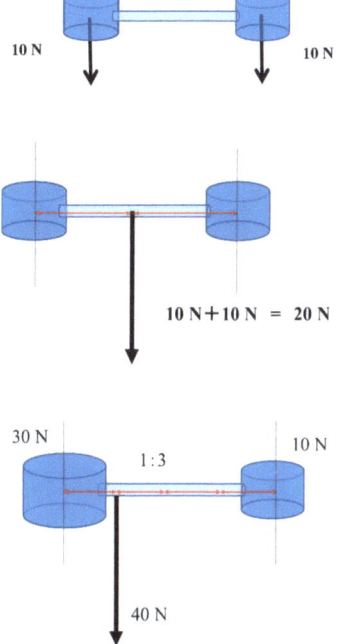

If the two forces are parallel but with different magnitudes, consider the line of action passing through the point of the reverse ratio of the magnitude of the forces.

For example, if the forces are 30 N and 10 N, the ratio of force is 3:1, and the ratio of distance is 1:3 through where the line of action passes. The magnitude of the resultant force will be the sum of the two forces, which is

30 N+10 N = 40 N.

This resultant force corresponds to the gravitational force acting on the center of gravity (COG) of the objects that are 3 kg and 1 kg connected, as shown in the figure (weight of the objects is 4 kg, so gravitational force is 40 N). The center of gravity is the point on which the actual resultant force of the gravitational forces applied to each object goes through.

Synthesis and Decomposition of Force

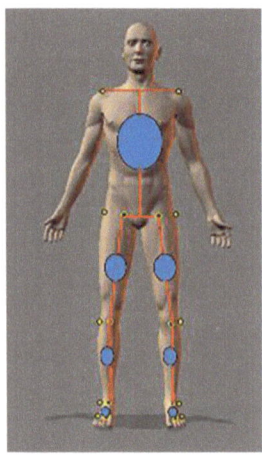

Application on the human body

Let's apply this idea to the human body. Consider the seven parts (segments) of the human body.

The gravitational force is applied to each segment's center of gravity. The sum of all these forces results in the center of gravity of the total body.

A combination of the seven gravitational forces will be applied to the COG of the entire body. The application point of this gravitational force applied to the whole body is called the COG of the entire body. The important point to remember here is that all of the forces exerted to each segment of the body are synthesized to one resultant force applied to the COG. Then, in this case, the human body can be replaced with a ball of the same weight as the body at the location of the COG of the whole body. Thus, the resultant force of a human body can be considered in the same way as the resultant force of a ball.

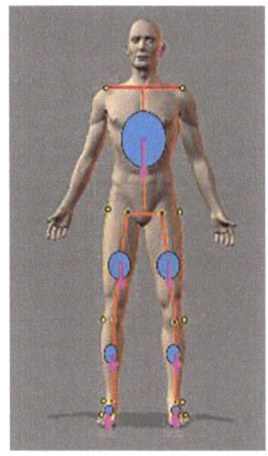

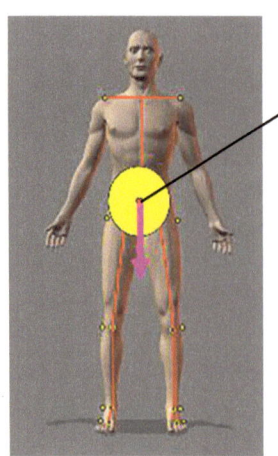

COG of the body
(same weight of the body as the ball)

Decomposition of force

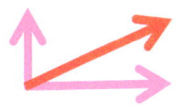

This time, contrary to the synthesis of force, let's consider the decomposition of force. Let's consider the force (red color) in the sagittal plane. This force can be decomposed in the horizontal and vertical directions. In synthesis, it is good to consider the diagonal of the two sides of the parallelogram. But now, imagine decomposing one force into two. The original force should be the diagonal of the rectangle made from the two forces.

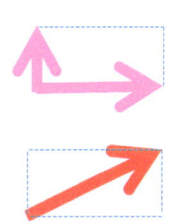

When decomposing one force into two, it is correct to use the parallelogram from the standpoint of mathematics. However, in basic biomechanics using the parallelogram is not recommended. Instead of using a parallelogram, please use a rectangle. As a rectangle is a type of parallelogram, it is mathematically correct to use a rectangle. Please remember to use the rectangle, as shown in this figure when decomposing forces in basic biomechanics.

Although we can see three forces in the above figure, it is essential to note that the three forces are not working at the same time. When the two decomposed forces (pink color) are working, the third force (red color) does not work because the third force is replaced by two forces.

Application on the human body
Force exerted on the spinal column

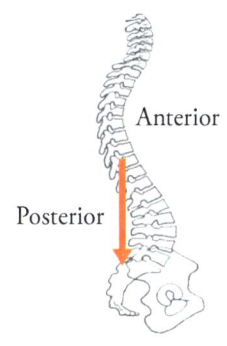

Focusing on some parts of the spinal column, the weight of the upper column exerting on the lower column is shown in the figure. Given that the weight of the upper side is 30 kg, the approximate gravitational force (orange) is 300 N.

Question: What are the compression force and shear force along the spine when you decompose this gravitational force?

Try to first answer this question by yourself.

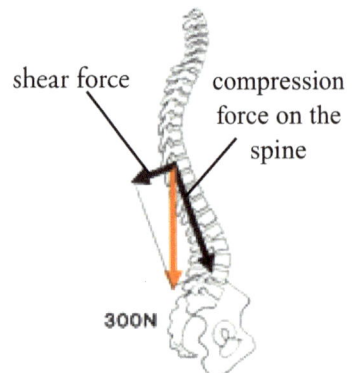

To consider the gravitational force as the diagonal, let's think about the rectangle as shown in the figure. The compression force applied to the spine will be smaller than the original gravitational force. Because the shear force is perpendicular to the direction of the spine, keep in mind that the shear force does not affect the compression force.

Example of the wrong decomposition

If you use a parallelogram instead of a rectangle, as shown in the figure, the force of 300 N will be considered as the diagonal of the parallelogram. The decomposition method itself is correct. However, such decomposition is inappropriate.

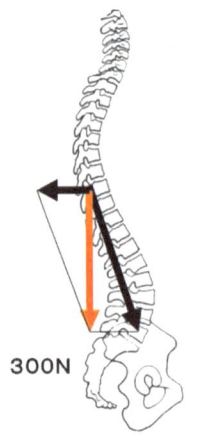

What if the spine is tilted more posteriorly? As you can guess from this figure, the force along the spinal column becomes much larger than in the figure. If the backward inclination of the spine is less than indicated in this figure, the force along the spine becomes smaller than the original orientation of the spine in this figure. In case the spinal column is vertical, the force along the spinal column will be 300 N, which is the same as the orig-inal force, and will be minimized. In other words, the more the trunk tilts backward, the higher the force exerted on the spine. However, such an explanation is wrong. The method of force decomposition is not illegal but the conclusion is incorrect.

Fundamental Biomechanics

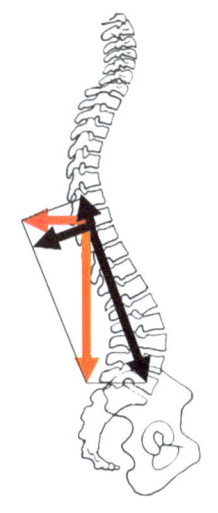

Why is the explanation wrong?
Please pay attention to the force in the horizontal direction. Horizontal forces (short red arrow) can also be broken down into two forces as shown by the two short black forces in the figure. The components of force along the spinal column were also hidden in the horizontal force. The hidden force has the reverse direction of the compression force. Thus, when we add this opposite hidden force to compression force, we will get a smaller force than 300 N, just as we showed the compression force when using the rectangle method. The gravitational force will not be adequately decomposed if you use the parallelogram method. This example has been previously described in some textbooks, however, just because it is written in textbooks does not necessarily mean it is correct.

Practice
Look at the figure. What percentage of the weight is applied to the sole, when a person is leaning on a tilting table? Here, cos (60°) is 0.5, sin (60°) is 0.87.

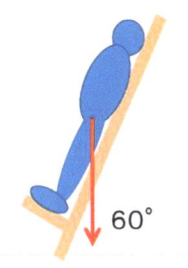

To solve this problem, we must first decompose the force. You can apply the correct answer as shown. Please be careful not to make an incorrect decomposition, as shown earlier in the example.

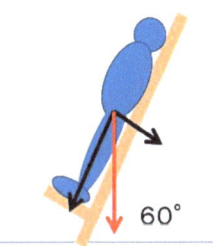

🖉 For teachers
Many students make mistakes here. Please let some students solve this question in front of a class and check.

Synthesis and Decomposition of Force

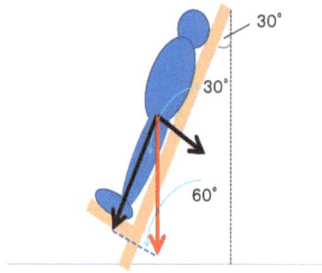

Let us consider the angle of the diagonal of the rectangle as shown in the figure. Since the inclination is 60°, the force perpendicular to the sole forms 30° from the vertical one.

The angle in the figure will be 60°.

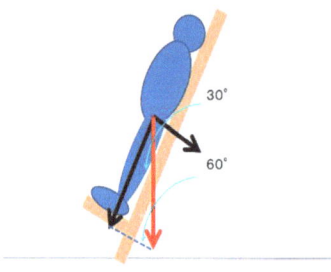

Note: The gravitational force was divided into two. The force applied to the sole will be 87% of the body weight, and the remaining force will be 50%. Even if the decomposed force is added directly, it will not become the original value because the two forces do not have the same direction.

Fundamental Biomechanics

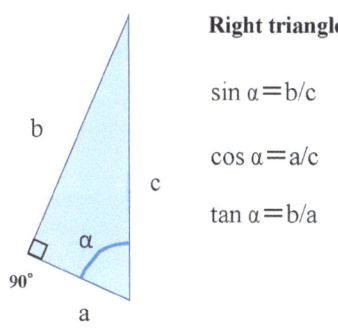

Right triangle

sin α = b/c

cos α = a/c

tan α = b/a

Let's review sine, cosine, and tangent in this example. Consider a right triangle as shown in the figure. Set the hypotenuse as **c**, the base as **a**, and the vertical side as **b**. At this time, the sin α is **b** divided by **c**, the cos α is **a** divided by **c**, and the tangent α is **b** divided by **a**. In the case of sine, the farthest side from the angle becomes a numerator, and in the case of cosine, the side that forms the angle with the hypotenuse becomes a numerator.

📋 For teachers
A considerable number of students have forgotten about sine, cosine, and tangent. Please take some time to practice.

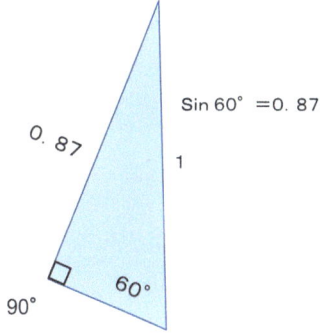

Sin 60° = 0.87

The figure shows the decomposition of the triangle. The lower right corner is 60°. The part of 1 corresponds to the weight of the subject. Since the component of force perpendicular to the sole is the furthest from the angle, we need to use the sine of the angle. Since the sin(60°) is 0.87, the component perpendicular to the sole becomes 0.87. Therefore, this component will be 87% of the weight of the person.

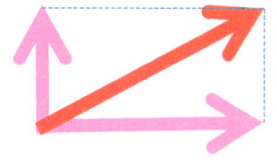

> **SUMMARY**
> In synthesizing forces, make a parallelogram whose two sides are constituted with the two forces. The diagonal becomes the resultant force. If the forces are parallel, the magnitude of the resultant force is the sum of the magnitude of the two forces. The line of action goes through a position close to the larger force. The way to decompose should be such that the original force is the diagonal of the rectangle.

CHAPTER 2

Applications of the Lever System to the Living Body

On completion of this chapter, you will be able:

1. To understand the lever systems
2. To understand the application methods of the lever systems on the human body

Many students may not have studied mechanics in high school. However, it is okay, because you have already learned about lever systems in science in the fifth grade of elementary school. Everyone knows lever systems well. However, just because you learned basic subjects in science, they cannot simply be applied to living bodies. The first necessary step therefore is for you to apply it to living bodies. You will learn this practice in this chapter.

Lever System

To make sure, let us review a fifth-grade elementary class on a lever system. What is the required force (kg) when the lever in the figure is balanced? You may solve this question with mental arithmetic; the length ratio is 4:1, so the weight ratio will be 1:4, and then the force will be 10 kg. Please never do such mental arithmetic.

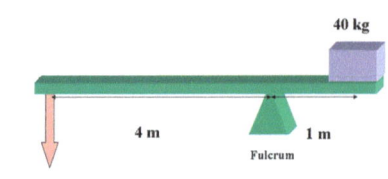

What is the force F for balancing?

Instead, make this kind of equation:

F kg × 4 m = 40 kg × 1 m. In this equation, F kg × 4 m should be set at the left side of the equation because F will rotate the lever system to turn left (counter-clockwise).

40 kg × 1 m should be set at the right side of the equation because 40 kg will rotate the lever to the right (clockwise). Make sure to attach units of **kg** and **m** (meter) at this time. Science is different from arithmetic. In mathematics, only numbers are handled, but in science, we deal with physical quantities, not numbers.

Our weight is 40 kg instead of 40. The length is 1m, not 1. When the equation like above is completed, calculate F kg.

F kg × 4 m = 40 kg × 1 m.

At this time, take 4 m on F to be the denominator on the right side.

Do not forget to attach the unit m (meter) here. Then, since there is unit m (meter) in the numerator and the denominator also has m (meter), these units can be reduced. As kg cannot be reduced, it remains as is. The answer will be 10 kg instead of 10. Here, the force of 10 kg times the length 4 m is called the moment of force. After all, the balance of the lever system means that the moment of the force of the left side is equal to the moment of the force of the right side of the equation.

Please solve next this problem below after you understand the lever system concept.
There is a weight of 60 kg at 1 m from the fulcrum.

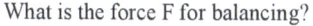

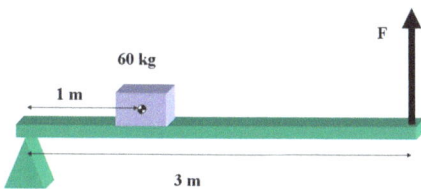

What is the force F (in kg) required to support this weight from the fulcrum?

60 kg × 1 m should be set at the right side of the equation because 60 kg will rotate the lever to the right (clockwise). Then, F × 3 m should be set at the left side of the equation because F will rotate the lever to the left (counter-clockwise).

📎 For teachers
Always let everyone write the moment formula and verify their answer. Please spend enough time until everyone can answer.

Please solve this problem. There is a weight of 60 kg at 3 m from the fulcrum. When force F is applied at 1 m from the fulcrum to maintain balance, how many kg is F?

F × 1 m should be set at the left side of the equation because F will rotate the lever to the left (counter-clockwise). Then, 60 kg × 3 m should be set at the right side of the equation because 60 kg will rotate the lever to the right (clockwise).

Applications of the Lever System to the Living Body

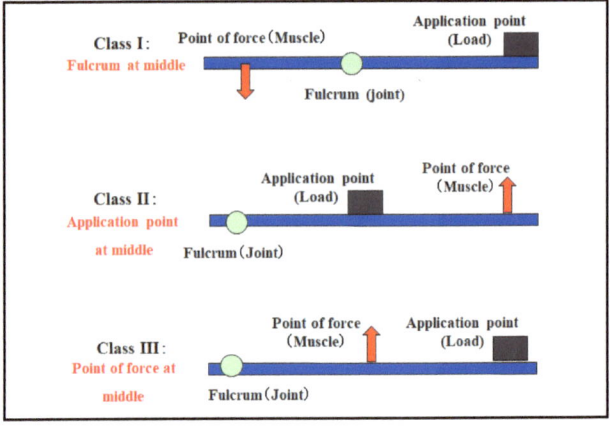

Let us summarize the three types of lever systems.

First, we term the lever system where the fulcrum is in the middle as a Class I lever system. Next, the lever where the application point occurs at the middle is called a Class II lever system. The application point may also be called the working point. Furthermore, when the point where the force is applied occurs in the middle it is called a Class III lever system.

In the case of a human body, please consider that the fulcrum is always a joint. The point of force is the attachment point of the muscle. The load point is the point where the weight can be put on.

Moment: Action of turning an object around a fulcrum with a force
- magnitude of force, force direction
- distance from the fulcrum (moment arm)

Moment of force = force magnitude × distance

Unit: Nm (Newton meter)

Revision of the lever system
Moment of force: The action of turning an object around a fulcrum with force. The magnitude of moment of force: it depends on force magnitude, the direction of force, distance from the fulcrum (moment arm).

Moment of force = force magnitude × distance (Unit is Nm)

Let us review the idea of the lever system again. The moment of force is referred to as the action of rotating an object around a fulcrum. The magnitude of the moment of force is determined by the magnitude and direction of the force and the distance from the fulcrum. Sometimes we call the distance from the fulcrum a moment arm or a lever arm.

The magnitude of the moment is "magnitude of force × distance".

Always measure the distance in a direction that is perpendicular to the force line from the fulcrum.

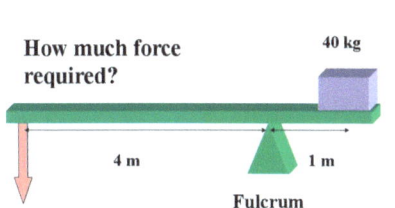

In the example above, we expressed force in kg to correspond with science in elementary school, but the formal unit of force is Newton (N).

For an object of 1 kg, please remember this is a force of 10 N (more exactly, 9.8 N).

Since the moment of force is the force multiplied by the distance, the unit is Nm (Newton-meters).

To be sure, let us practice using the Newton (N) units. When the lever in the figure is balanced, how much force is required? (The answer is displayed on the bottom of the next page)

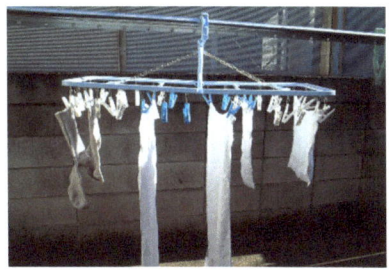

For teachers
As an example of a lever system, please explain the equilibrium of a rack for laundry. We already know about the balance of forces when using a rack for laundry. Please also describe the force that supports the weight of the whole laundry.

Applications of the Lever System to the Living Body

Tips for applying to a living body

What does the term "Lever" mean?

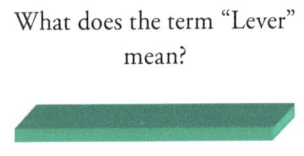

What is the term "Lever"?

Now that a review of the lever system is complete, its application on the living body will be explained. That is, to better understand what the lever system is referring to in the living body.

What part is a lever?
The lever is the stick in the figure.
When the lever system is applied to the living body, the lever is not shaped like a stick. It is important to correctly determine which parts of the body correspond to this lever. Practice is then necessary for that.
Unfortunately, this practice is not done at elementary school. From now on, the application on the human body will be explained.

Let's practice a little before entering the main subject.
Please write the force of the 40 kg block as an arrow on the lever in the example of the previous lever system. Try solving this assignment by yourself.

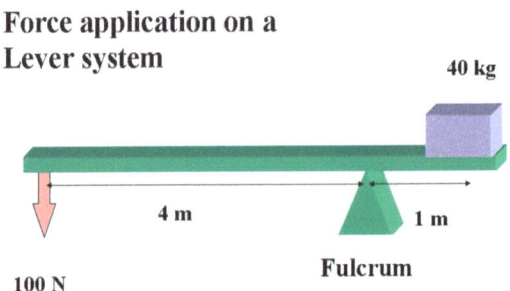

(Response from the previous page)
F × 4 m = 400 N × 1 m, and the answer is 100 N.

Fundamental Biomechanics

Force application on a lever system

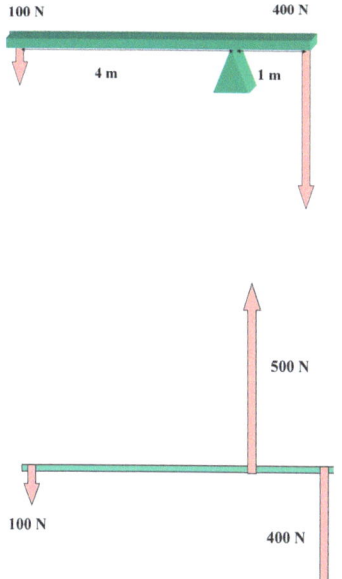

This is the correct answer.

How much is the force on the fulcrum?

Since the lever receives both 400 N force and 100 N force at the fulcrum, there is a total of 500 N on the fulcrum force as shown in the figure.

The first important point is that the force applied to the lever system from the fulcrum is opposite in direction to the other forces. The second important point is that the three forces cancel each other and become zero when the three forces are added as you can guess by looking at the figure.

This is true for any lever system when the system is not moving. Please do not forget, because these are important points.

Now, let us perform some practice applications. Which part is the lever in the figure? The forearm and hand (combined) represent the lever. The elbow joint is the fulcrum. The part where the biceps brachial muscle is attached to the forearm is the point where the force is applied. The location of the gravity of the teapot represents the action point (load point). Next, draw the forces on the lever as arrows at the load point and the application point. Please try to solve this assignment before moving to the next page.

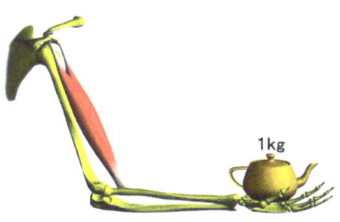

From Human Anatomy for CG creators

Applications of the Lever System to the Living Body

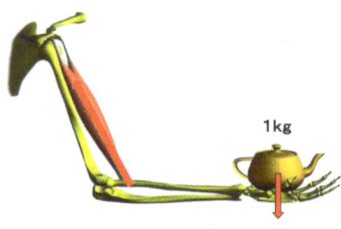

It is wrong to draw the force that applies to the teapot, as shown in this figure. In this case, the force represents the gravity on the teapot. Instead, you should draw the forces applied on the lever. Where is the lever? The lever is the forearm and the hand, not the teapot. That is the reason why I asked you which part of the body is a lever.

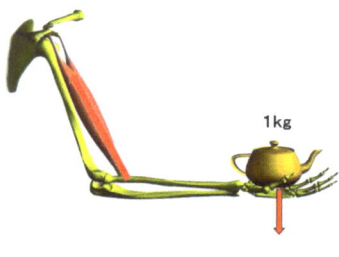

This is the correct answer.

How much force F should the muscle apply to hold the teapot in place? The fulcrum is the elbow joint. Since the force acting on the action point of the hand is vertical to the horizon, the distance from the fulcrum to the force of 10 N should be measured horizontally. Let this distance be 30 cm. The line of action of the biceps brachii muscle is inclined from the vertical line. Therefore, a perpendicular line is drawn from the elbow to the line of action. Note that it is not on the horizontal line. Let this distance be 5 cm.

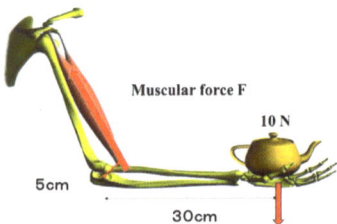

The formula becomes

$F \times 5 \text{ cm} = 10 \text{ N} \times 30 \text{ cm}$,

then force F = 60 N.

Here the force required for the muscle is larger than the gravitational force of the teapot.

Fundamental Biomechanics

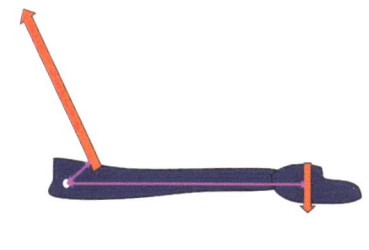

If you extract only the lever system and draw it, it will look like this figure. Here the force required for the muscle is larger than the gravitational force of the teapot. Like this case, in a living body, the lever often demands greater force. Usually, the lever uses a small force to generate a large force. On the contrary, the lever in the living body reduces the large force into a small force.

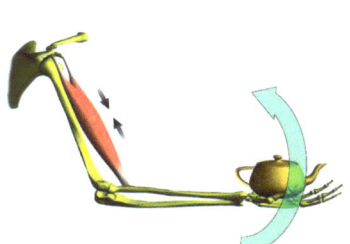

Then, what is the advantage of this lever system? Please look at this figure. The range of motion of the hand is very large. Instead of requiring six times the amount of force, you can get up to six times the range of motion with a slight shortening of the muscle. At the same time, it also means that the speed at the force point is expanded six times faster at the application point. This fundamental biomechanical construct is evident in nature, when animals need to quickly escape from a predator or catch prey. This lever becomes the third lever with its point of action in the center.

A person of 60 kg weight stands on one leg. How much force is required for the triceps surae?

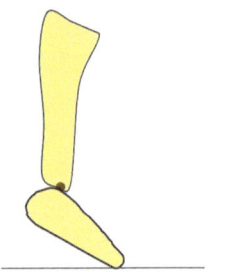

Application to the lower limb

Now, let's apply the lever to the lower limbs of the body. A person of 60 kg is tiptoeing with one foot. What force is required for the triceps surae? First of all, we need to figure out which part of this figure is the lever.

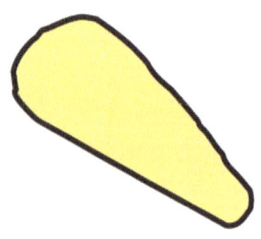

When the foot is considered as one stick, the foot becomes the lever.

The ankle joint becomes the fulcrum of the lever.

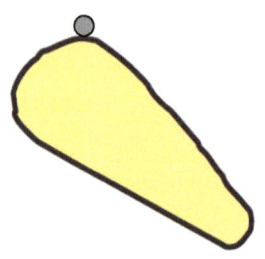

Next, think about where the fulcrum is. The ankle joint is the fulcrum and in living bodies, joints are the fulcrums.

Let us determine the load point.

Since the floor reaction force is applied to the toe, that is the load point.

Let the distance from the fulcrum to the load point be 20 cm. The key is to remember that the distance from the fulcrum is to be measured orthogonally to the line of action of the force. In this case, the floor reaction force acts vertically to the floor, so measure the distance from the fulcrum horizontally.

Finally, let us consider a force point. The force point is the attachment part of the triceps surae muscle. The distance from the fulcrum (ankle joint) to the force point is 5 cm, as shown in this figure.

Once we have determined the force point of the triceps surae and the floor reaction force, we can calculate the force F of the triceps surae muscle.

$$600 \text{ N} \times 20 \text{ cm} = F \times 5 \text{ cm}$$

$$\therefore F = 600 \text{ N} \times 20 \text{ cm} / 5 \text{ cm} = 2400 \text{ N}$$

It should be noted here that the muscular strength required for the triceps surae muscle is four times the weight of the body. Some reference texts say that the triceps surae muscle requires forces less than the bodyweight while tiptoeing. However, this is incorrect, and is an example of a misdirected application of dynamics.

How much force will be applied to the joint (fulcrum)?

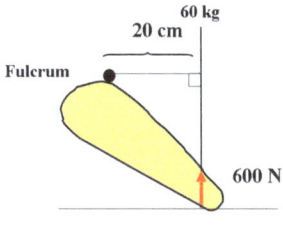

A person of 60 kg stands on one leg. How much is the force F? (Strength of the triceps surae)

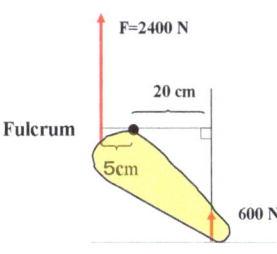

How much force will be applied to the joint (fulcrum)?

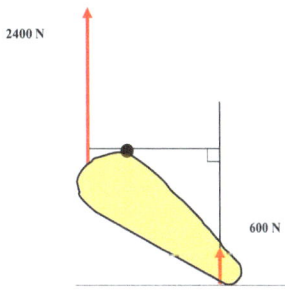

Applications of the Lever System to the Living Body

📝 For teachers

Please take time to solve this assignment. Please let the students consult each other for discussion.

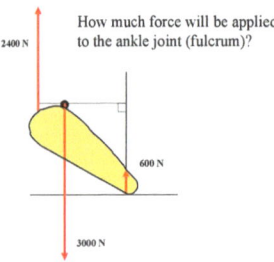

How much force will be applied to the ankle joint (fulcrum)?

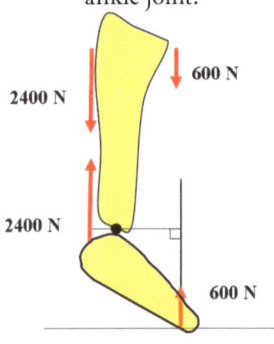

Not only 600 N but also 2,400 N is added to the ankle joint.

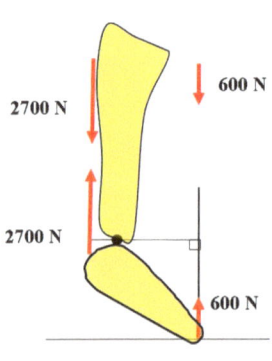

Answer

The fulcrum will bear 3,000 N totaling 2,400 N and 600 N. As learned before, adding all three forces on the lever system will cancel each other out to zero. You should be able to answer this.

However, you may not be convinced that the ankle joint bears five times the weight of your body. However, thinking carefully, there is already the gravity of 600 N on the body above the ankle in the first place. Here, the weight of the foot part is not taken into consideration because it is light. To the Achilles tendon, the triceps surae exerts 2,400 N force, pulling the heel up. Of course, since the origin of the triceps surae is above the ankle joint, it pulled down the body with a force of 2,400 N. The ankle must withstand both of these forces. Therefore, 3,000N is applied.

The more the application point moves forward, the more triceps surae muscle strength is required. The joint force also increases. The more the weight moves towards the toes, as shown in the figure, the more force needed for the muscles and the inter-joint force also increases at the same time. Remember that such high forces are exerted on joints during normal walking. The shank and the feet are mutually exerting their forces. This force is transmitted primarily by the joint (through bone to bone) and the muscles.

Of these forces, the force transmitted through bone to bone is called the inter-joint force. A force of 3,000 N is applied downward from the shank, which is the joint force. On the other hand, 2,400 N of force is applied upward through the muscles. It means that a total force of

600 N is transmitted from the shank to the foot. Naturally, a force of 600 N is applied in the opposite direction from the foot to the shank. This force is called the intersegment penetration force.

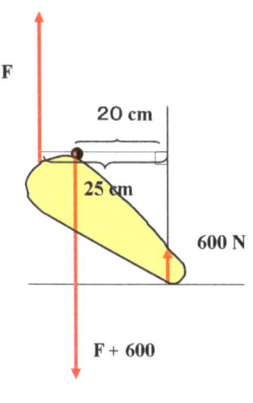

For teachers

When thinking about the lever system, there is also a way to think of the toe as the fulcrum of the lever. In other words, the foot is considered as a second-class lever, and in this case, it is mistakenly thought that the force applied to the ankle is 600 N.

As can be seen in this figure, the force applied to the ankle joint is the sum of the body weight and the force F of the triceps surae. In this case considering the toe as fulcrum, the equilibrium equation is as follows:

(F + 600 N) x 20 cm = F x 25 cm. You can sort out this equation to calculate F.

F x 20 cm + 600 N x 20 cm = F x 25 cm

F x (25 cm – 20 cm) = 600 N x 20 cm

F= 2400 N.

You can get the correct answer even if you consider the toe or ankle as fulcrum.

SUMMARY
It is important to determine which part of the living body represents a lever system and think about the forces applied to that lever system.

CHAPTER 3

Center of Gravity (COG) calculation

On completion of this chapter, you will be able:

1. To explain lever systems
2. To explain the concept of the center of gravity
3. To explain how to calculate the center of gravity
4. To understand how a change of posture affects the center of gravity

Everyone knows the phrase center of gravity (COG). However, few people understand it correctly. Being able to explain the center of gravity correctly is the first item of order towards an understanding of biomechanics applications.

Center of Gravity (COG) calculation

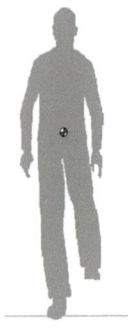

Revision of the lever system
1)   How much is the force of the gluteus medius muscle?
2)   How much is the force applied to the hip joint?

Let us do additional exercises on revision of the lever system.

Let us think about the muscular strength necessary for the gluteus medius muscle and the supporting force at the hip joint while standing with one leg. First, in this example, where is the lever considered to be? Here, the hip joint force is the force applied to the hip joint, which is the fulcrum.

For teachers
I think it is quite a challenge for students. Please take time to assist students.

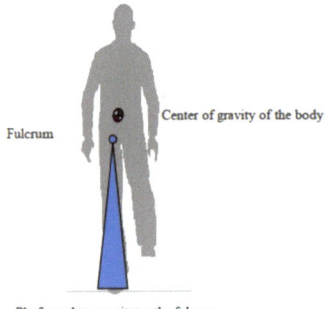

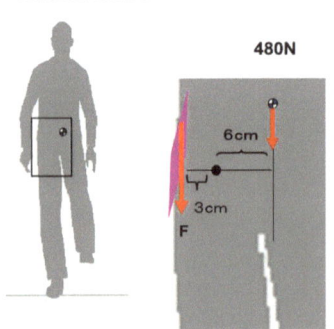

Let us consider the bodyweight except for the weight of the standing leg. The hip joint represents the fulcrum. In other words, let us think that the hip joint as a fulcrum supports the weight of the upper body (upper body + one lifted leg on the other side). The center of gravity (load point) of the "upper body + one leg of lifted side" was written in the figure (load point).

The horizontal distance between this center of gravity and the hip joint is 6 cm. The mass of the "upper body + one leg of lifted side" is about 80% of the body weight.

Here we set it to 48 kg. In other words, the gravitational force is 480 N. One key component of this lever is where the gluteus medius attaches to the pelvis. Let's set the horizontal distance between the hip joint (fulcrum) and the attached point of the gluteus medius to be 3 cm. Assume that the gluteus medius muscle pulls vertically.

As a reference, the weight ratio of the body parts is about 60% for the upper body and about 20% for one leg.

Fundamental Biomechanics

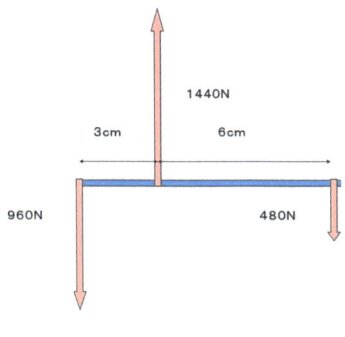

You can then calculate the force of the gluteus medius muscle to be 960 N and the inter-joint force to be 1,440 N.

Here, is it not strange that an upward force is applied at the hip joint? You may think that the direction of the force should be downward. This force is upward because it is the force that the lever receives at the hip joint. Conversely, a downward force is applied to the base which constitutes the fulcrum.

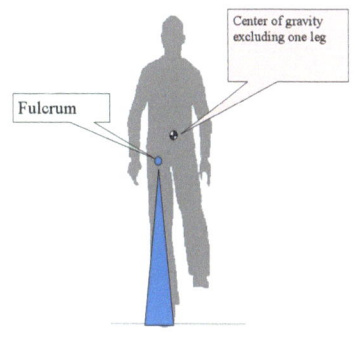

Let's think about the center of gravity of the body when standing on one leg. The hip joint represents the fulcrum. Do you have any doubts concerning this? Do you think it is necessary to consider the right side and left side separately? Because the mass on the left side tilts the body "to the left" and the mass on the right side tilts the body "to the right".

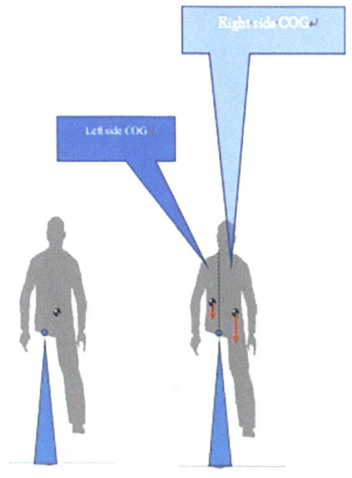

Do not worry.

Considering the fulcrum separately, the center of gravity only on the right side is more to the right than in the previous figure. The left part is on the left side of the fulcrum. The center of gravity combines these two points, that is, the center of gravity of the body, excluding the support legs is shown in the previous figure. When thinking about the center of gravity of an object like this, you can think that all of the mass of the object is concentrated at the center of gravity.

Center of Gravity (COG) calculation

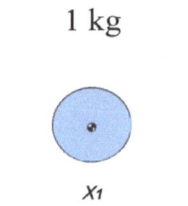

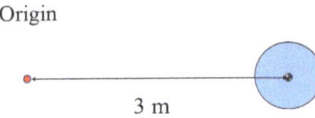

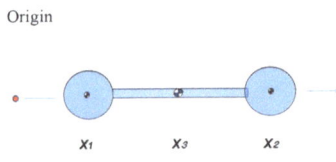

Determination of COG

Let's consider how to calculate the location of the center of gravity. The center of the ball represents the center of gravity and we assume the ball is made with a uniformly distributed material. If the coordinate of the center of the ball is x_1, then the coordinate of the center of gravity is x_1.

If the origin is set at 3 m in order to indicate the COG, the value of 3 m will be the coordinate of the center of gravity position.

Now let us consider the center of gravity when two objects are connected. The center of gravity of the bar connecting two spheres of the same mass is the midpoint of the line connecting the centers of the two spheres. Let's express this with a mathematical formula.

Suppose that ball No. 1 with a mass of 1 kg is at x_1 position and that ball No. 2 is a mass of 1 kg at x_2. When the two balls are connected by a bar, the coordinates of the center of gravity can be expressed as follows: $x_3 = (x_1 + x_2) / 2$.

The equation above shows the middle point of spheres No. 1 and No. 2 locations. If the two spheres are at 3 m and 4 m, then $x_1 = 3$ m, $x_2 = 4$ m,
$x_3 = (3 \text{ m} + 4 \text{ m}) / 2 = 3.5$ m, then x_3 is the average of 3 m and 4 m ($x_3 = 3.5$ m).

What if the masses of the two balls are different? Suppose the respective masses of balls 1 and 2 are 1 kg and 3 kg.

Consider the center of gravity of the object connecting these two balls.

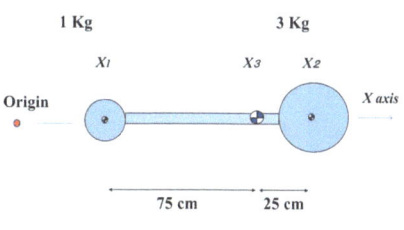

Assuming that the distance between X_1 and X_2 is 1 m, 3/4 of the length from the location of No. 1 to the location of No. 2 is the location of the center of gravity. The center of gravity is 75 cm away from X_1.

Now, let's consider this object as a seesaw. At first, suppose the object is supported just below the center of gravity. The center of gravity is at a distance of 25 cm from ball No. 2, so this position represents the fulcrum. The following equation can be set: on the right side, 3 kg x 25 cm; on the left side, 1 kg x 75 cm, where the left side = right side and the equation's balance is maintained. Next, suppose the object is not supported below the center of gravity. In this case, the equation's balance is not maintained.

When the center of gravity is used as a fulcrum like this, the balance of the lever system is maintained. In other words, the position where the balance of masses can be maintained can be considered as the center of gravity. Let's consider the following example also with a formula.

Let's assume that ball No. 1 with a mass of 1 kg is in the position of X_1, and the ball with a weight of 3 kg is in the position of X_2. When these two balls are connected, the coordinates of the center of gravity can be expressed as follows.

$$X_3 = X_1 + (X_2 - X_1) \times (3/4)$$

Therefore

$$X_3 = (1/4) X_1 + (3/4) X_2$$

The total mass of balls No. 1 and No. 2 is 4 kg. Therefore, the denominator of the coefficient in the above equation is 4. The numerator 1 of the coefficient for X_1 corresponds to 1 kg of ball No. 1. The numerator 3 of the coefficient for X_2 corresponds to the weight of 3 kg of ball No. 2. In other words, the center of gravity can be considered as a weighted average value with the mass of the objects that make up the part as the "weight".

Center of Gravity (COG) calculation

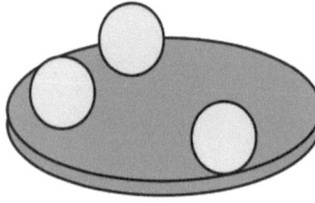

3 balls on a tray

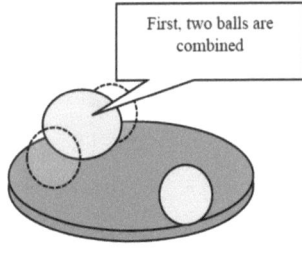

First, two balls are combined

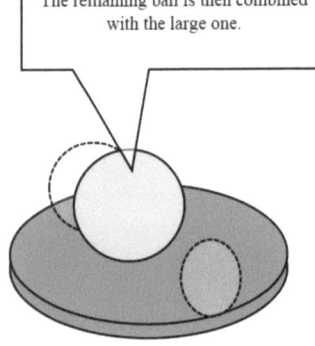

The remaining ball is then combined with the large one.

Observe the example above in which the balls are aligned in a straight line (it is natural because of the two balls). Still, a similar equation can be applied even if the three balls are not in a straight line.

For example, as shown in this figure, let's suppose that three balls are placed on the tray. Assume the tray has no weight.

It can be understood that the position of the center of gravity of the whole tray changes depending on the arrangement of the balls.

In this case, first, determine the COG of the two balls.

The center of gravity of the whole tray can be found by combining the large ball with the remaining third ball.

In this case, please note that the mass of the three balls will be combined to the total center of gravity.

Fundamental Biomechanics

First calculate the joint center position from the markers attached to the body surface.

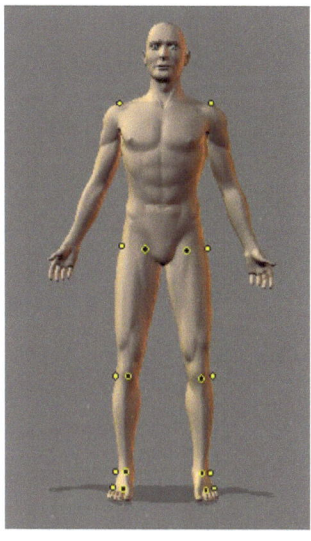

Here the head, trunk, arms, and pelvis represent one segment.

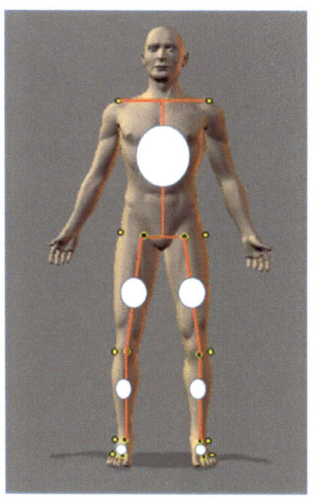

COG of the human body

Now, let's determine the center of gravity of the body. For the sake of simplicity, the head, trunk, arms, and pelvis are considered as one body segment. Using the attached reflective markers to the body surface, we can measure the position of the markers with a motion capture camera. Motion capture cameras are devices that acquire human motion through use of a computer.

This system is used for making computer graphics for movies (cinema) and motion of characters of video games. Next, we can calculate the joint center position from the markers.

Let's assume that the center of gravity of the segment is on the line connecting the joint centers. The position of the center of gravity of the segment can be calculated by measuring the marker position. Suppose that the center of gravity of the body segment is on the line connecting the joint centers. The specific parameter is based on the value obtained from the anatomical body. In this way, if you determine the marker position, you can calculate the center of gravity of the segment. Thinking this way, we can replace the body with seven balls. In other words, the same ball as the mass of the segment exists at the center of gravity of each segment of the body.

Center of Gravity (COG) calculation

Next, the center of gravity of each ball will be synthesized sequentially.

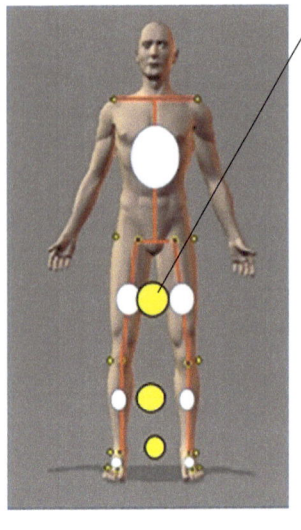
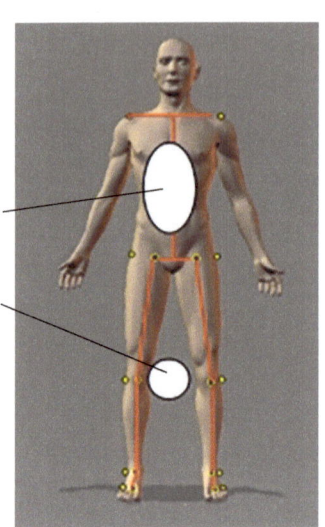

Combination of right and left thigh

Combination of upper body COG

Combination of lower limbs COG

Now you get two balls, as shown in the figure. It can be called the upper center of gravity and lower center of gravity. Roughly, the mass ratio of upper body and lower body is 6 and 4 respectively.

In the end, we will have one ball. The final (red) ball represents the center of the gravity of the body. The mass of the ball is the same as the mass of the whole body.

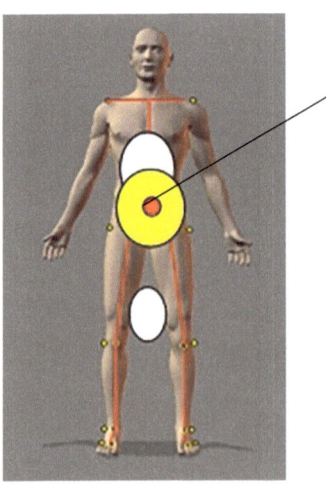

Center of gravity of the Body
(The red ball has the same weight as the body mass)

Thus, the combined center of gravity of the seven balls represents the COG of the body. If the position of the COG of segments changes, the total COG moves inside or sometimes outside of the body. For example, in a standing position, the COG is located at about 53% of the body height measured from the floor to the middle of the pelvis (in front of the sacrum). However, it is not necessarily located in the central part of the pelvis. For example, when sitting, holding the knee, or a back-stretching posture, the COG will not be in front of the pelvis.

The relation between the ground reaction force and the center of gravity
As a good example, the animation shows the relationship between the ground reaction force and the center of gravity in the standing position. You can see how the ground reaction force supports the center of gravity.

In the second example, let's observe an animation. The center of gravity in the sitting position is different from the standing position.

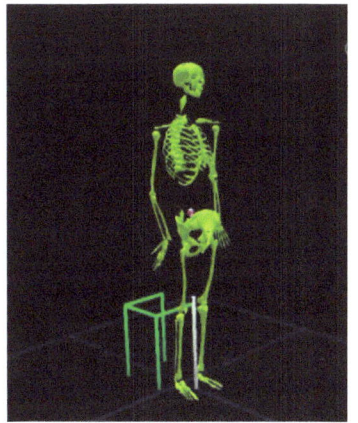

> **SUMMARY**
> The position of the center of gravity depends on body posture.

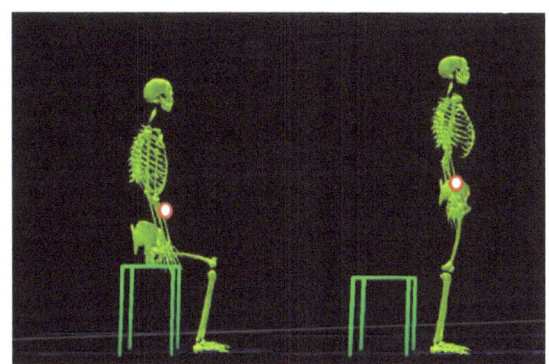

CHAPTER 4

Velocity and Acceleration of the Center of Gravity

On completion of this chapter, you will be able:

1. To explain the velocity of the center of gravity
2. To explain the acceleration of the center of gravity
3. To draw a graph of the velocity of the center of gravity when standing up and sitting down
4. To draw a graph of the acceleration of the center of gravity when standing up and sitting down

Squat movement

From the upright position, think about the action of bending the knee and squatting while keeping the upper body upright.

At this time, draw a graph of the vertical position of the center of gravity, that is, the change in height of the center of gravity with time.

📎 For teachers

Please demonstrate the squat movement as follows: from the upright position, bend the knee to about 45° and hold this posture for 3 seconds.

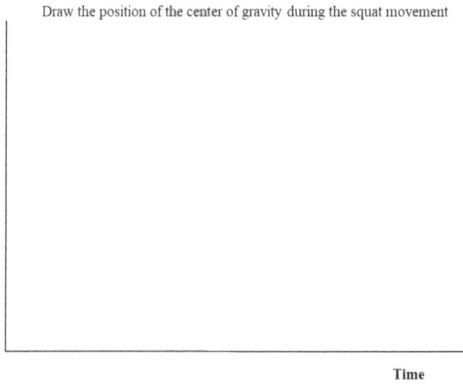

Draw the position of the center of gravity during the squat movement

Next, draw the graph of the vertical velocity of the center of gravity.

📎 For teachers

Please demonstrate the same squat movement as shown earlier.

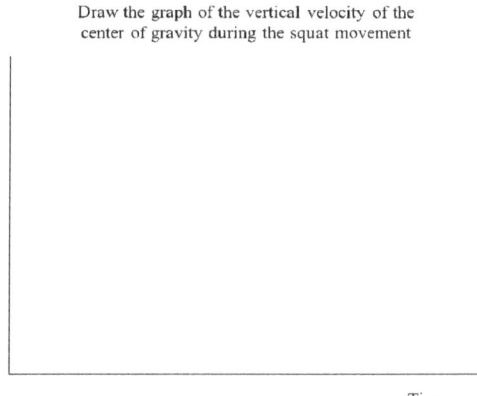

Draw the graph of the vertical velocity of the center of gravity during the squat movement

Fundamental Biomechanics

Draw the vertical acceleration of the center of gravity during the squat movement

Time

Next, draw the graph of the vertical acceleration of the center of gravity, focusing on the vertical movement during the squat movement.

🔧 For teachers

Please demonstrate the same squat movement, as shown earlier. Most students might not be capable of drawing a graph of acceleration.

What is acceleration? (Please ask the class)

Acceleration is the amount of velocity that increases or decreases within one second. In general, acceleration is not constant during one second. So, it is difficult to calculate the amount of velocity that increases or decreases in one second. Therefore, in this case, think of acceleration as follows: Let's say there is a 5 m/s increase in velocity for 0.1 seconds, while assuming that the same acceleration continues for 1 second, the velocity will be 50 m/s. Acceleration is an amount that indicates how much the velocity will increase in one second. The value obtained by multiplying the increment of 0.1 seconds by 10 is the acceleration. When the velocity decreases, the decrease is indicated with a minus sign. Imagine a scene where you start driving a car. If you press the accelerator, the speed will increase. If you gradually press more on the accelerator, the speed will increase gradually. When the maximum velocity is reached, the velocity does not increase no matter how much the accelerator is pressed. In other words, the acceleration is zero. There is no acceleration while driving at maximum velocity. If you apply the brake, the velocity will decrease. At this time, the acceleration is negative. If you continue to apply the brakes, the car will stop. While this car stops, the velocity is zero, and the acceleration is also zero.

Use this knowledge and draw the vertical acceleration of the center of gravity during the squat movement.

📎 For teachers

Please ask three students to draw graphs on the blackboard at the same time.

Please indicate this model solution on the blackboard and correct the student's answer.

- It is necessary to include the static data before the movement.
- It is necessary to include the static data after the movement.
- The connecting part at rest and the movement should be round.
- At the end of the movement, the graph should be round.
- Please insert vertical lines at the start and end of the movement.

Height of the center of gravity during the squat movement

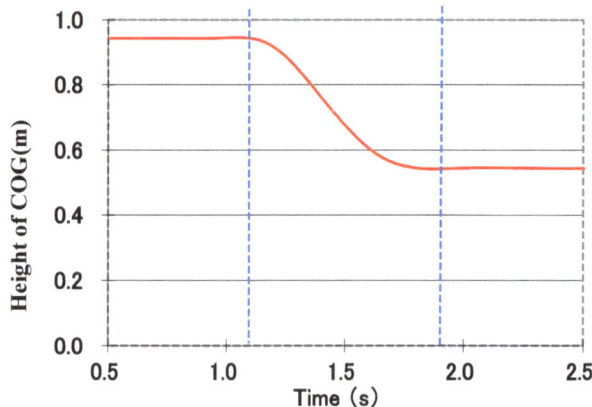

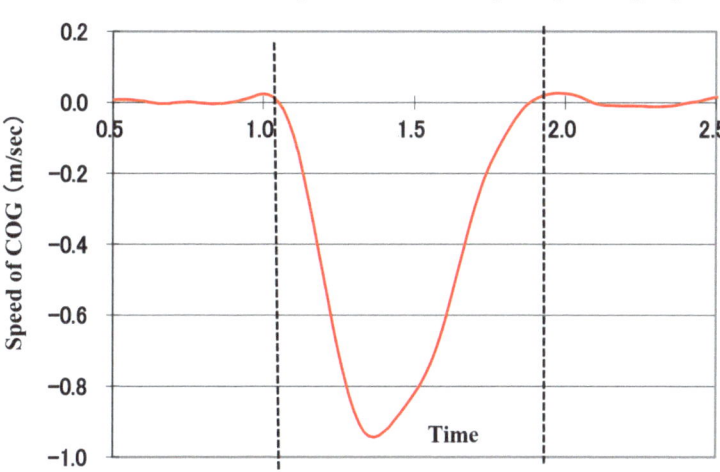

📎 For teachers

Assign at least three students to draw the graph of the velocity of center of gravity (COG) on the blackboard at the same time.

Indicate the model solution on the blackboard and correct the student's answer.

- The timing should be the same as the graph of the height of the center of gravity.
- Please insert vertical lines at the start and end of the squat movement.
- The velocity should be negative. (Most students make a mistake)
- The connecting part at rest and at the time of movement should be round.
- At the end of the movement, the graph should be round.

In activities of daily life, the velocity of rising and velocity of descent may be considered positive values as well. However, in biomechanics, it is very confusing when we use positive values for both rising and descending movements. Therefore, coordinate axes are set in three directions: anteroposterior, mediolateral, and vertical. The velocity is assumed to be positive if the velocity is the same direction as the coordinate axis; the reverse direction is considered negative. For example, if the coordinate direction is positive from Tokyo to Osaka, the velocity of the Shinkansen (bullet train) going from Tokyo to

Osaka will be positive, and conversely, the velocity of the Shinkansen going from Osaka to Tokyo will be negative.

In the case of the squat movement, the higher the position of the center of gravity in the first graph, the greater the value. At this point, the vertical coordinate axis is implicitly determined to be positive upward. Therefore, the upward velocity is positive, and the downward velocity is negative. So, the correct answer is negative, as shown in this graph. By the way, in biomechanics, we use the word "speed" to express a distance per second without considering the direction of the movement. So, speed always has a positive value. Speed is a scale of the Shinkansen speedometer. Speedometer does not have a negative value. Velocity is a distance per second considering the direction of movement. There is a distinction between positive and negative in velocity, and there is no distinction between positive and negative in speed. Therefore, in activities of daily life, we should use the word "speed", not "velocity". You may consider the absolute value of velocity as speed. The unit of velocity is m / s (meter per second, travel distance per second).

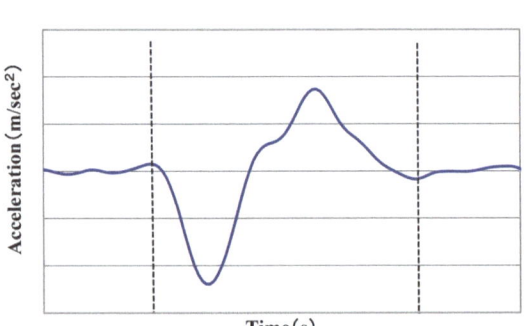

Acceleration of COG graph during the squat movement

📋 **For teachers**

Assign three students to draw a graph of the acceleration of the COG on the blackboard at the same time.

Please correct it strictly.

- The timing of the acceleration graph should be the same as the graph of the height of the COG.
- Please insert vertical lines at the start and end of the squat movement.

- The first half is negative acceleration, and the second half is positive acceleration.
- The point where the acceleration is zero coincides with the point of negative velocity peaking at the middle point of the movement.
- The connecting part from rest to start of movement should be round.
- The area of the negative part should be equal to the area of the positive part.

In the first half of the movement, the negative velocity increases, so the acceleration becomes negative. In the second half of the movement, the negative velocity decreases. Therefore, the acceleration becomes positive. At the middle point of the movement, the acceleration is zero because the negative velocity is highest at the midpoint of the movement.

In the case of movement that starts from static and ends at static like the squat movement, the area of the positive and negative parts of the acceleration must be equal. When the area of positive acceleration is not equal to the area of negative acceleration, the velocity cannot return to zero. The unit of acceleration is m / s² (meters per second squared).

Relationship between COG, velocity, and acceleration

Relationship between COG, velocity, and acceleration

Let's arrange three graphs vertically: height of COG, velocity, and acceleration. These three graphs are closely related to each other. First, observe the height of COG and the velocity graphs. You can draw the graph of velocity just by looking at the graph of the height of COG. Let's think about how to do this correctly.

Let's think of the change in height on the graph as a side view of the roller coaster rail. Let's put a box on this rail. The incline of this box corresponds to the velocity. When at a stationary position, the box is horizontal. At this time, the velocity is zero. As time progresses, think of the box in the second position on the COG height graph. The box tilts to the lower right side at the start of the movement. Downslope corresponds to negative velocity. Negative velocity increases. Eventually, the slope of the rail will be maximum at the midpoint, and of course, the box will have the largest downward angle. The third box is the maximum negative velocity. After the midpoint, the slope becomes horizontal. The velocity approaches zero and eventually becomes zero. In this way, the angle of inclination of the box corresponds to the velocity.

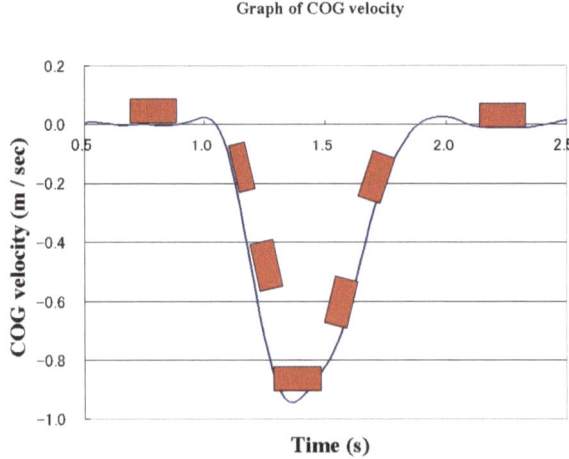

Similarly, if the graph of velocity is assumed to be the rail, then the incline angle of the box corresponds to the acceleration. In the first half, the slope falls to the right side, so the acceleration is negative. At the midpoint, the box will be horizontal for a moment. At this time, the acceleration is zero. In the second half, the slope is upward to the right. At this time, the acceleration is positive. Gradually, the slope becomes horizontal and acceleration becomes zero.

Fundamental Biomechanics

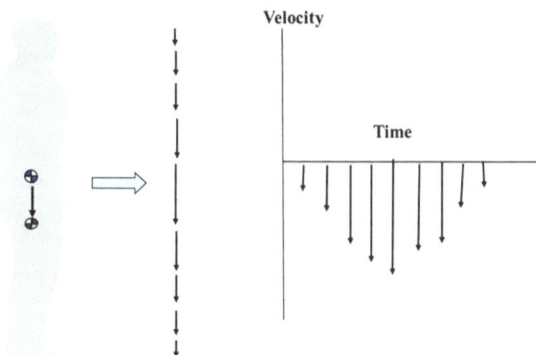

📝 For teachers

While the center of gravity during the squat is moving downward, students might have doubts that the acceleration will be positive. In this case, please explain as follows:

Let's look at the movement of the center of gravity during a squat with time division. At the beginning, the COG is moving slowly, then fast and then slow. The arrows on the graph become the graph of velocity by arranging these arrows side by side on the horizontal time axis.

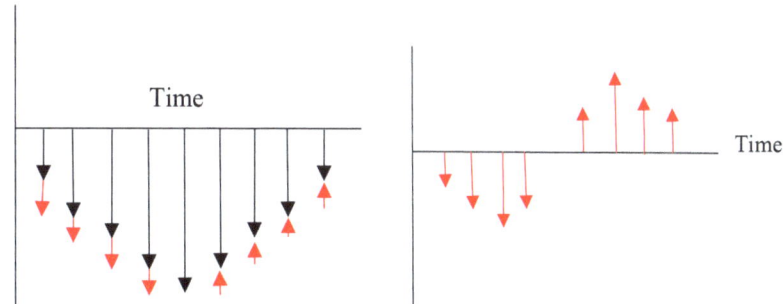

At first, the black downward arrows gradually become large. At the middle of the time course, the downward black arrows become maximal and then decrease to finally become zero at the end of the movement. The difference between one arrow and the next arrow is the acceleration. In this graph, the red arrows represent the acceleration. In the first half of the time course, the red arrows are downward. In the second half of the time course, the red arrows become upward. The red arrows become the graph of acceleration by arranging these arrows side by side on the horizontal axis. However, the arrows in this explanation are just conceptual diagrams, and the actual velocity and acceleration are the amount of change per second.

Standing up from the sitting position

For practice, try drawing the graph of the COG height, velocity, and acceleration when you stand up from the sitting position. These figures show the model solution for the graphs during rising from a chair.

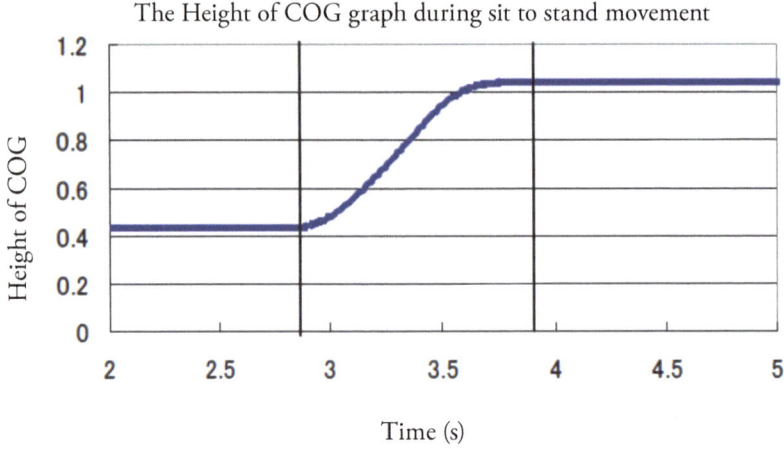

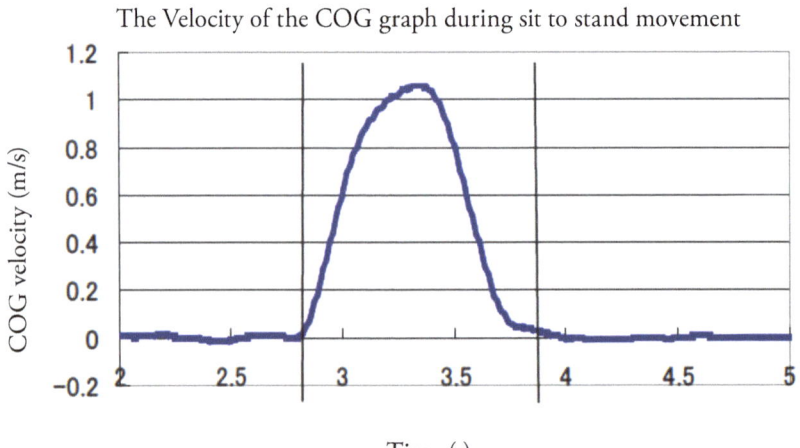

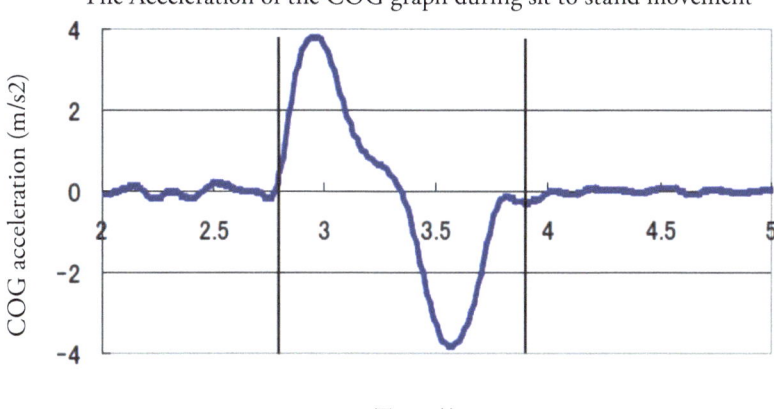

The Acceleration of the COG graph during sit to stand movement

SUMMARY

The velocity of the COG and the direction of acceleration are not the same.

Acceleration depends on the change of velocity, therefore: the positive acceleration has the effect of accelerating the upward movement. Also, the positive acceleration has the effect of decelerating the downward motion. The negative acceleration has the effect of accelerating downward and decelerating while moving up. The theory of acceleration may not be easy to understand. However, the acceleration of the COG is important because it is closely related to the dynamics of the ground reaction force. Please understand it.

CHAPTER 5

Ground Reaction Force and COG Acceleration

On completion of this chapter, you will be able:

1. To explain the relationship between the force and the acceleration of the COG
2. To explain the ground reaction force exerted on the body
3. To explain the relationship between the ground reaction force and the movement of the COG during squatting

You have already learned about force and acceleration of the COG. You will learn about the relationship between these two subjects. First, let's study the general theory.

Ground Reaction Force and COG Acceleration

Let's think about the relationship between the movement of COG of a ball and the force.

🛍 For teachers
In the first part of this chapter, don't let the students open the textbook. Please explain only with a PowerPoint. Focus on the center of gravity of the soccer ball and consider the relationship between movement and force.

Force and acceleration of COG
Let's suppose that the ball starts moving from the left side. Please neglect gravity.

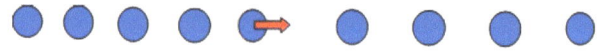

Application of force

Suppose that the force acts for a short period on the ball while it is flying. The red arrow represents the force. The force acts only for a short time, and it disappears immediately. When it disappears, the arrow also disappears. How does the state of the ball change?

🛍 For teachers
Please assign a student to answer.

Model answer:
  The velocity of the ball increases. Moreover, the increase in velocity is only during the period when the force is acting. When the action of the force is over, the increase in velocity is also over. However, the increased velocity is maintained.

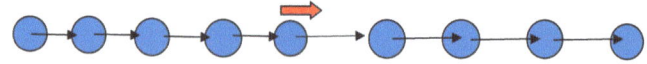

Application of force

Let's observe once more. This time, the force and velocity are shown. The black arrow represents the velocity. When the force is not applied, the length of the black arrows is constant. The force is represented by the red arrow. The velocity increases because the force is applied. Even if the application of force is over, the increased velocity remains.

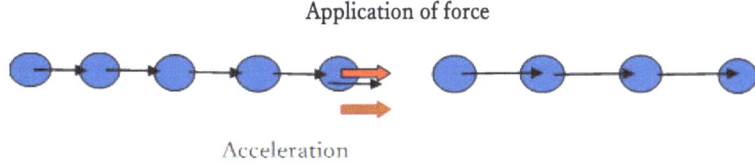

Application of force

Acceleration

Acceleration occurs when there is a force

Let's observe again the figure above. This time, acceleration is added. The orange arrow represents acceleration. The force is applied in the middle of the course and simultaneously the acceleration occurs. You can notice that the velocity increases. As soon as the force is over, the acceleration is also over.

Force produces acceleration

The acceleration (α) and the force (F) are proportional.

α = F / M

(M is the mass of the ball in kg)

This indicates that the acceleration and the force arrows are in the same place and in the same direction.

Force produces acceleration
When the force is applied, the object is accelerated. Acceleration is proportional to the force.
 Also, if the mass of the ball is large, less acceleration will occur. The acceleration will be inversely proportional to the mass of the object.
 The equation formula will be α = F / M
 If this equation is shown graphically, we can observe that the acceleration and the force arrows are pointing in the same direction as shown in the figure above.

Ground Reaction Force and COG Acceleration

How is the force exerted on the human body when standing on the ground?

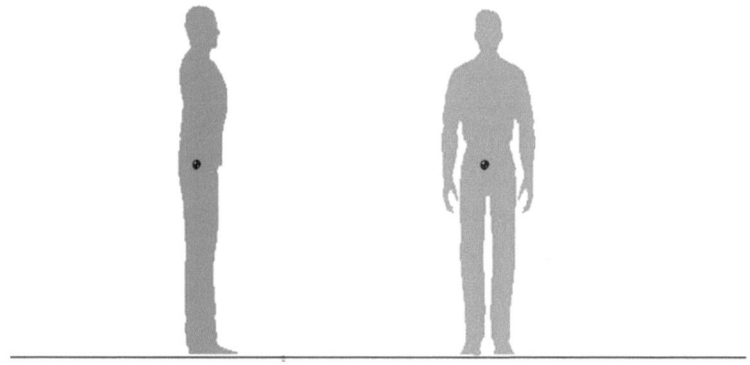

When force is applied, acceleration occurs on the object. This is a general theory of the relationship between force and acceleration. This applies to the human body as well. First, let's consider the force applied to the human body. How is the force acting on this person when they are standing on the floor? Please draw the force in the figure above.

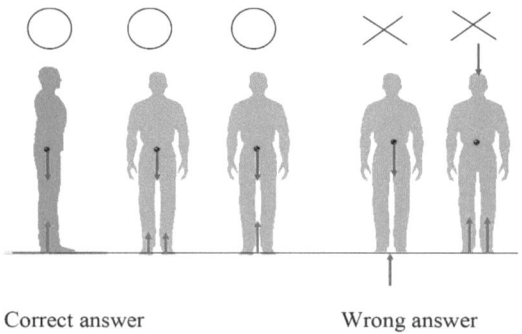

Correct answer   Wrong answer

📝 For Teachers

Please ask three students to draw the force exerting on the body on the blackboard.

- Even if you write the ground reaction (GRF) force on the left and right legs, it is OK. However, the sum of the "magnitude" of the GRF on the left and right leg should be equal to the magnitude of the gravitational force.

- Please write the ground reaction force arrow so that it comes out from the floor.
- It is wrong to draw the arrow of the ground reaction force under the floor.

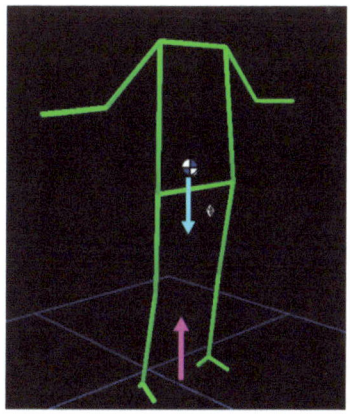

Gravitational force and the ground reaction force act on the body when standing on the ground.

Gravity and the Ground Reaction Force

Gravity and the GRF act on the person standing on the floor. The GRF acts on the left and right legs. To understand easily the relationship between the force and the movement of the human body, the left and right ground reaction forces were combined into one as shown earlier. Now you can observe something interesting. What do you observe? (Please let the students answer.)

Gravity and GRFs are the same in magnitude, opposite in direction and on the same straight line. The gravity and the GRFs cancel each other, and their sum equals zero. In other words, "No force is acting on the human body when standing on the floor." Because the force is not acting, it can be standing still. In daily living activities, we always feel that there is a reaction from the floor. However, the GRF is canceled by gravity from the point of view of biomechanics. Gravity has always acted the same way since we were born, so we don't usually feel it.

Ground Reaction Force and COG Acceleration

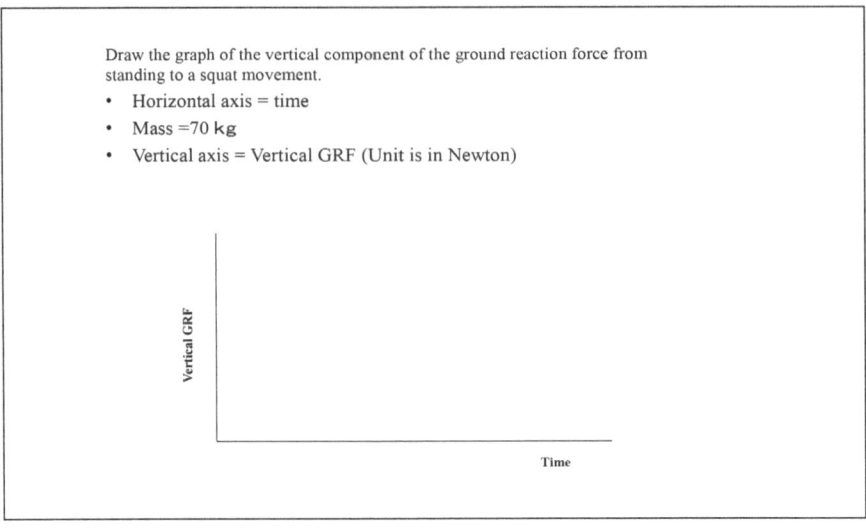

Keeping in mind the situation mentioned above, consider the case where a person standing on the floor performs a squat movement. Draw the graph of the vertical component of the GRF from standing to a squat movement.

📝 For teachers

Demonstrate the squat movement by bending your knees from an upright position. Assignment: Draw the graph of the vertical component of the GRF when the knee is bent and squatted from an upright position. The horizontal axis is time. Mass is 70 kg. The unit of the vertical axis is N (Newton).

📝 For teachers

In some cases, please bring a weight scale to the classroom and use it. Put the scale on the floor and let one student stand on it. The student's mass appears on the scale. If the mass is 70 kg, the vertical component of GRF is approximately 700 N. When standing still, the vertical component of the GRF is constant. Please observe the value of the weight scale when the student performs a squat movement on the scale.

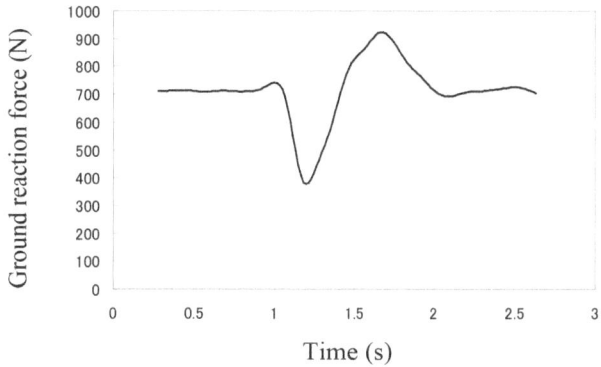

🗒 For teachers

Please designate three students to draw the graph on the blackboard. If it is drawn as shown in the figure, it is correct. It may not be easy to draw. Please give time for the students to discuss between each other. Please compare the GRF graph with the graph of acceleration at squat drawn in the previous chapter. You will see that the previous graph and the current graph look the same. The graph of the previous acceleration is decreasing and increasing around zero. In the case of the GRF, the value decreases and increases around 700 N. Although the value itself is different, the tendency to decrease, increase and return is the same. There are good reasons for this. This is the relation between the GRF and acceleration. In this situation, the force is the sum of the gravitational force and GRF. In this way, the acceleration of COG and the sum of gravitational and GRF is proportional.

🗒 For teachers

Although this graph also has a slight fluctuation of the waveform, the model solution should be the graph of the textbook.

For a better explanation, look at the following:

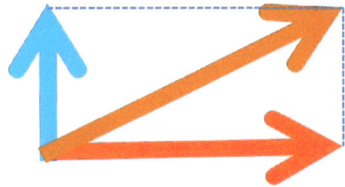

When considering force and movement of an object, it is fundamental to identify the mediolateral, anteroposterior and vertical force components. As shown in the figure, the force acting diagonally is displayed separately in the anteroposterior direction and the vertical direction. The force was projected on the Y and Z axes. Although not shown in the figure, the mediolateral direction (X-axis) can be displayed as well. When projected in this way, the three shadows that were projected are called "components of the original vector". Specifically, it is called the mediolateral direction component, the anteroposterior direction component, and the vertical direction component.

These components correspond to the mediolateral, anteroposterior, and vertical directions. Each can be expressed by a single numerical value. For example, the anteroposterior component can be expressed as 200 N. At this time, special treatment is applied to the sign of the number. If the component's direction is the same as the coordinate axis, the component's numerical value is expressed as positive, and if it is opposite to the coordinate axis, it is expressed as negative.

For example, if the upward coordinate axis in the vertical direction is positive, the upward component is expressed as +300 N, etc. The gravity applied to an object weighing 1 kg is approximately 10 N, but since the direction of the gravity is opposite to the Z-axis, the vertical component of gravity is expressed as -10 N. You might be wondering, "What is a negative force?" The force vector is not negative, but only the component values can be expressed as negative.

If you take the coordinate axis downward in the vertical direction, the component of gravity will be + 10 N, not -10 N. It's just a matter of definition.

The gravity acting on the COG always points directly downward. Assuming a mass of 70 kg, the vertical component of gravity is -700 N. The components in the anteroposterior and in mediolateral direction are zero. As for the GRF, the vertical direction is always upward, so it has a positive value, and the value changes momentarily during movement. The anteroposterior and mediolateral components change with time while becoming positive or negative. Since the major movement of a squat is up and down movement, we will consider the vertical components of gravity and the GRF.

If the vertical component of the GRF is expressed as Wz, the GRF is always upward, so Wz is positive. On the other hand, since gravity is downward, it is expressed as -700 N. If you sum both, it will be Wz-700 N (Please read N as Newton). This force exerts on the person standing on the floor.

The mass of this person was 70 kg, so dividing the force by the mass gives the acceleration. Let αz be the acceleration of the COG:

$$\alpha z = Fz / M$$
$$= (Wz-700 \text{ N}) / 70 \text{ kg}$$

αz: Vertical component of the COG acceleration
Fz: Vertical component of force applied to the human body
Wz: Vertical component of the GRF
M: mass

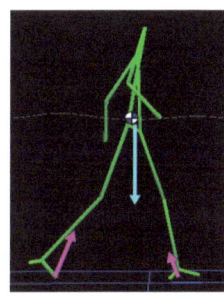

Vertical component of the ground reaction force on a body standing on the floor

Wz -700 N
Wz: vertical GRF

Acceleration calculated from the GRF

- $\alpha z = Fz / M$
- $= (Wz-700 \text{ N}) / 70 \text{ kg}$

- αz: Vertical component of the center of gravity acceleration
- Fz: Vertical component of force applied to the human body
- Wz: Vertical component of floor reaction force
- M: mass

This is Newton's law of motion. Since Wz is the ground reaction force, this equation expresses the relationship between the ground reaction force and the acceleration of the center of gravity. That is, you can calculate the acceleration by subtracting 700 N from the ground reaction force and dividing it by 70 kg. If you subtract and divide with constant numbers, the results themselves will change, but the shape of the graph will not change. Therefore, the graph of acceleration and the graph of the GRF will be similar.

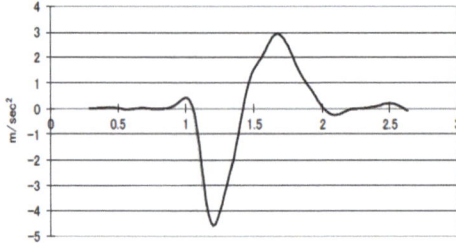

Acceleration calculated from the Ground Reaction Force

This is the acceleration of the center of gravity calculated from the ground reaction force. The acceleration was calculated by subtracting 700 N from the GRF and dividing by 70 kg.

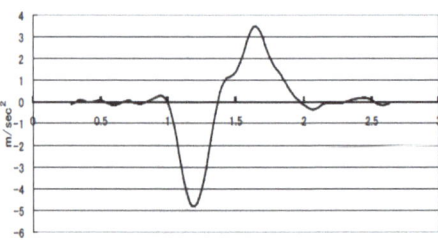

Center of Gravity Acceleration calculated from the position of COG

This is the acceleration calculated from the COG position measured by motion capture cameras.

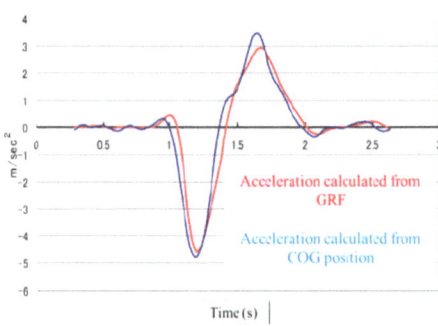

Let's overlap and display the above two graphs. There are some differences in the details, but it can be seen that they almost overlap. Thus, we can see that the GRF force corresponds to the acceleration of the COG.

Fundamental Biomechanics

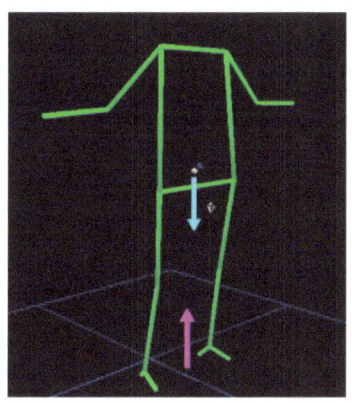

Let's explain this again with illustrations. When standing upright, gravity and ground reaction force cancel out, and the total force applied to the body is zero. Therefore, the center of gravity does not have acceleration and remains stationary.

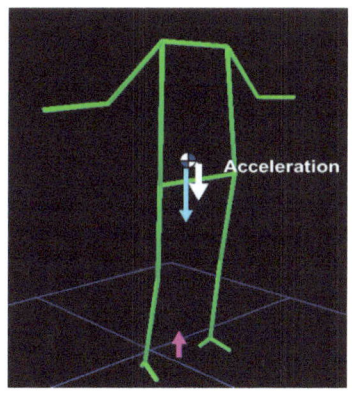

When the reaction force is smaller than gravity, the downward force is generated by the amount of subtraction. Therefore, the downward acceleration is generated at the center of gravity according to this.

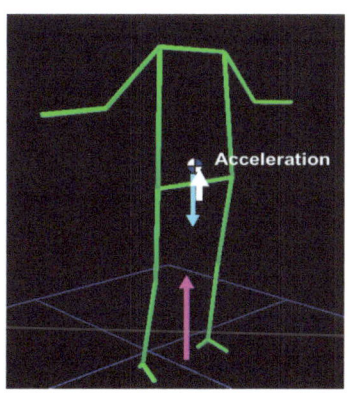

If the ground reaction force is greater than gravity, an upward force will appear by the amount of the difference. Therefore, the center of gravity has an upward acceleration according to this force.

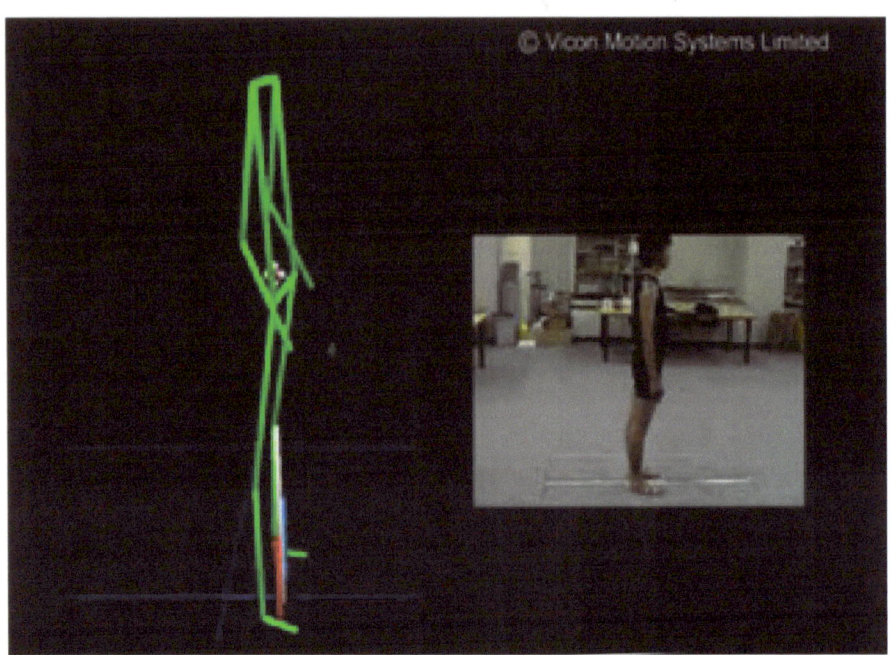

Finally, let's observe the ground reaction force when performing a squat movement from a standing position. You can observe that the ground reaction force first decreases, then increases and finally returns to its original value. Next, let's observe when we rise from a sitting position. You can observe it getting bigger, smaller, and returning to its original value.

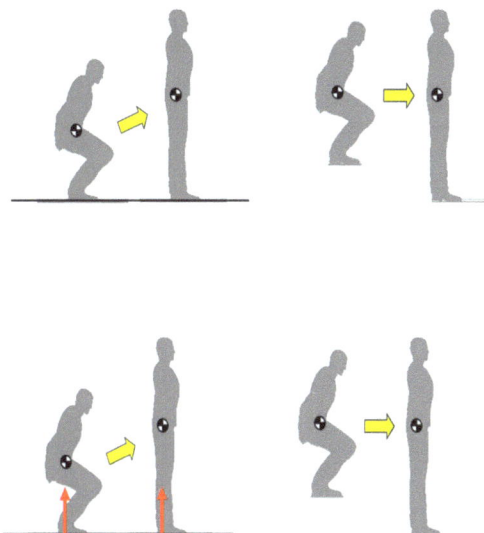

Muscular Force and Ground Reaction Force

You have learned that the GRF and the acceleration of the COG correspond to each other. At first glance, it seems that the COG moves because there is a GRF, but this is not the case. The driving force that moves the body is muscle strength. Think about the relationship between muscle strength and the GRF. What will happen if you activate the extensor muscles of the knee from the state of squatting down on the floor to standing upright as shown in the left figure? The knee extends and the COG rises upward. The figure on the right side shows the same thing in space on a spacecraft. If you activate the extensor muscles of the knee, the knee will extend, but the position of the COG does not change.

What is the difference between the two? In the figure on the left, the activity of the extensor muscles of the knees causes the feet to press the floor and generates the reaction force. The GRF moves the center of gravity upward. Within a spacecraft (figure on the right), there is no reaction force caused by the extension of the knee joint because the feet do not contact the floor. Therefore, the center of gravity does not change even if the knees extend. Thus, the driving force of the movement is muscle activity, but in a spacecraft, muscle strength is used only to move "segments". To move the center of gravity as well as the "body segment", the ground reaction force is necessary.

SUMMARY
The change of the acceleration of the COG is due to the presence of the GRF.

CHAPTER 6

Center of Pressure (COP)

On completion of this chapter, you will be able:

1. To explain the meaning of center of pressure
2. To explain the relationship between center of pressure and base of support
3. To explain the relationship between the center of pressure and the center of gravity position
4. To explain the character of the center of gravity, the ground reaction force and the center of pressure during standing, sitting, and reaching movements

The Center of Pressure is the point of application of the ground reaction force. What exactly is center of pressure? Since it is a very important term in biomechanics, please understand it properly.

Center of Pressure (COP)

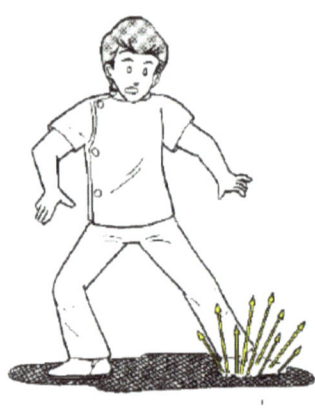

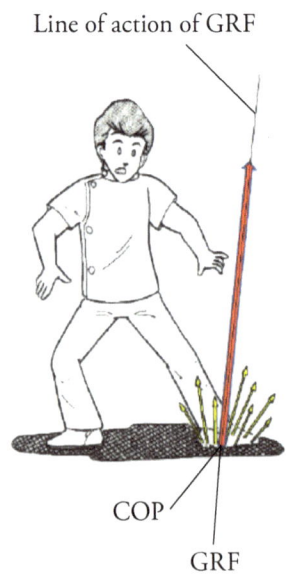

Line of action of GRF

COP

GRF

Center of pressure definition

When the foot comes in contact with the floor, there are always reaction forces at the contact area as shown in the figure. The reaction forces in each part varies in magnitude. The directions are also different.

The reaction forces in each part may be parallel to one another or may be in different directions. In any case, the reaction force is certainly upward. The reaction force is not pointing downward. We already learned that multiple forces can be combined, and as shown in the figure, the reaction forces distributed in the sole of the foot can be combined into one force. In the figure, only the reaction of the left foot is displayed, but the reaction of the right foot can be displayed in the same way. The force drawn in red at this time is called the ground reaction force (GRF). In this example, the location where the ground reaction force should be displayed depends on the distribution of the reaction force. Because the reaction force is synthesized, the position of the synthesized force is fixed at a certain point. As we learned in the synthesis of forces, the "position" in this case is the "position of the line of action". Although the position of the line of action of the synthesized force is known, it does not matter where on this action line the force is displayed. It may be displayed anywhere on the action line. Therefore, for the sake of convenience, the ground reaction force is typically displayed on the floor surface. The base point of the ground reaction force is called the application point of the ground reaction force, or the center of pressure (COP).

Fundamental Biomechanics

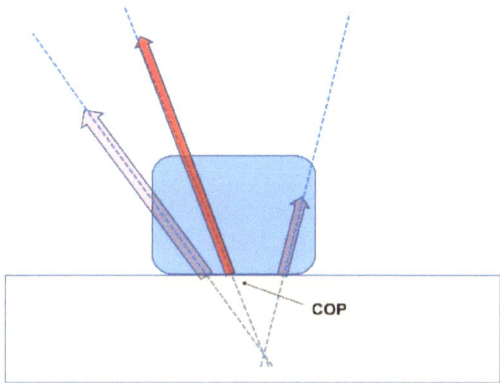

Let's review the synthesis of force. From the figure, let's combine the two pink forces. If you move the pink forces along each of their action lines to the intersection point and make a parallelogram, the diagonal red force will be the combined force. The resultant force moves along the diagonal, starting from the floor surface of the object, as shown in the figure. In this example, the position of the base of the red arrow is the COP. Thinking this way, COP does not have the original pink forces acting on it. The COP may be at a different location than where the forces do work. The COP is a location where the virtual combined force acts.

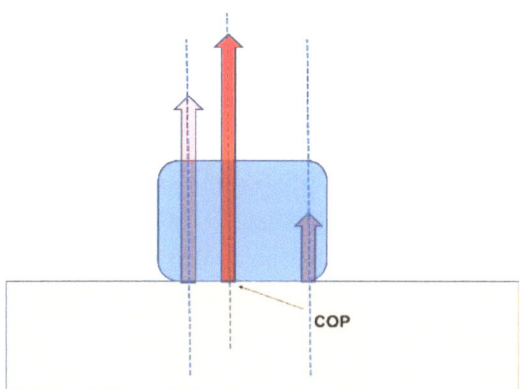

Let's review the case when the original forces are parallel to each other. The magnitude of the combined force is the sum of both forces. The line of action of the combined force is determined by the size of the original forces. The combined force location is closer to the larger force. Even in this case, the COP is located where the pink original forces do not apply.

65

Center of Pressure (COP)

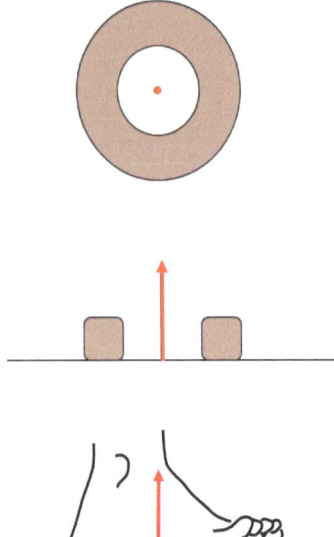

The COP is at a place where the foot is not in contact with the floor

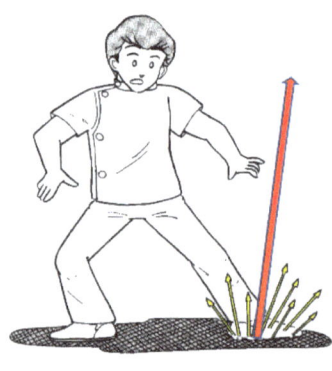

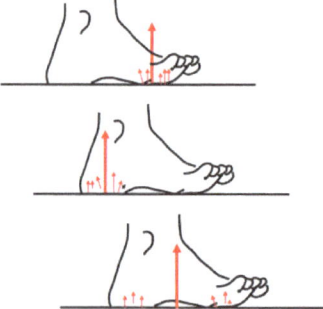

For example, when a donut is placed on a plate, the combined point of the reaction force from the plate is at the point where there is no donut. If you think about a person standing on a floor, COP may be located in a place where the foot is not in contact with the floor. An example is a case where the COP is positioned at the arch of the foot.

As explained so far, the ground reaction force is a collection of all the reaction forces distributed in the feet. The sum of the vertical components of the reaction force is the vertical component of the ground reaction force. The sum of the mediolateral and anteroposterior components of the reaction force is the mediolateral and anteroposterior components of the ground reaction force, respectively. COP is the average position of distributed reaction forces. Intuitively, the COP may come near the largest reaction force, but this is not always the case, because COP is determined by the distribution of reaction forces over the entire foot sole.

Therefore, if most of the reaction forces are distributed to the toe, COP will be located on the toe. If most of the reaction forces are distributed in the rearfoot, the COP will be in the rearfoot. If the reaction forces are distributed in half at the forefoot and at the rearfoot, the COP is located in the arch. The position of COP depends on the distribution of the ground reaction forces.

Fundamental Biomechanics

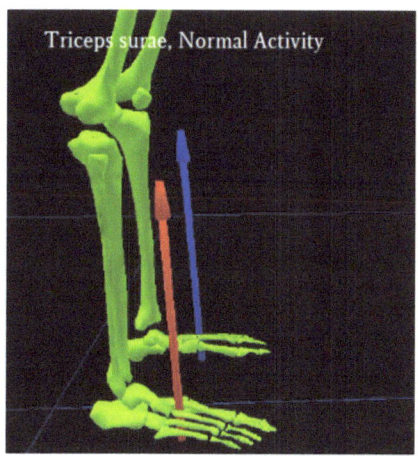 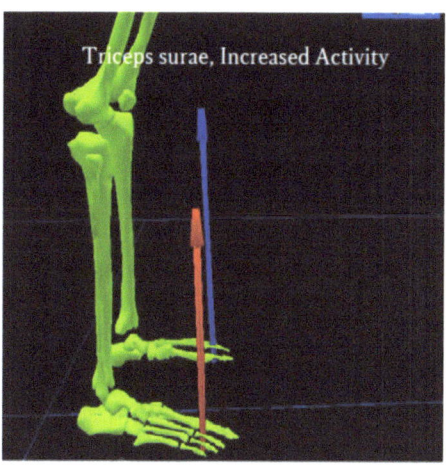

COP during standing. The left figure shows a normal condition. The right figure illustrates moving the center of gravity to the toe side.

Let's consider the COP during standing. The figure on the left is a normal standing position. You can see that the COP is in the midpoint for both the left and right foot. At the same time, we can see that the COP is anterior to the ankle. Although not shown in the figure, the component of the combined COP is approximately in the middle of the left and right COPs, and the COG is directly above the combined COP. In this way, if you know the position of the COP at rest, you can know the position of the center of gravity in the mediolateral and anteroposterior directions. Also, COP is in front of the ankle joint, which indicates that the triceps surae muscle is active. This can be better understood by learning joint moments. Joint moments are learned in Chapter 7.

The figure on the right shows the case where the center of gravity is shifted to the toes. COP also moves to the toes in response to the movement of the center of gravity. The fact that the COP moves closer to the toes also means that the ground reaction force moves away from the ankle joint. In such a case, it is expressed that the activity of the triceps surae muscle is greater than before. By observing the COP, the state of muscle activity can be imagined. If the movement is slow, the center of gravity is directly above COP, so you can find the approximate position of the center of gravity. However, since COP is a position on the floor, the height of the center of gravity cannot be known through this method. Thus, COP is important data that must be analyzed through motion analysis.

Center of Pressure (COP)

COP and Base of Support

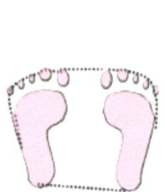
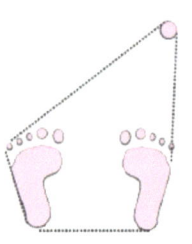

Cane

The COP can move within the range of the base of support.

When stationary, the COG is above the base of support. Let's consider the COG and the COP together. The base of support can be thought of as the range within which the COP can move. In the standing position, the COP is the point of action of the combined forces of the left and right feet ground reaction forces. When you are using a cane, COP is the point of action of the combined forces of the left and right feet and the cane.

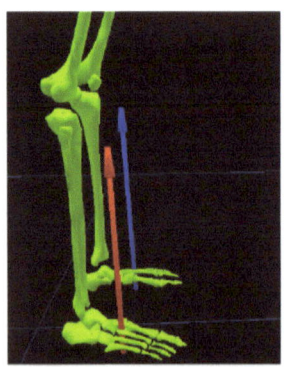

Let's observe again the standing position. When standing, ground reaction forces are acting on the right foot and left foot.

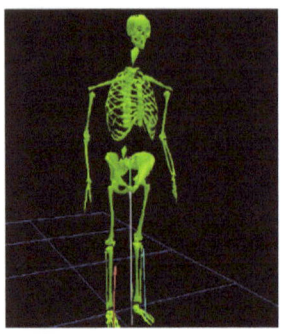

If you combine these forces into one ground reaction force, you can see that the combined ground reaction force indicated by the white arrow is directly below the COG.

Fundamental Biomechanics

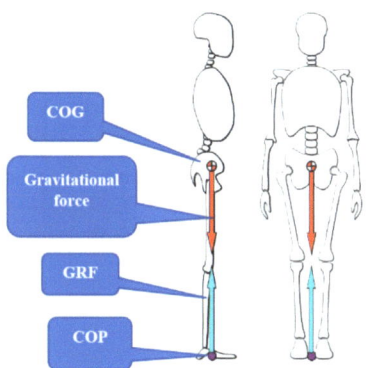

The gravitationale force is acting on the COG. When standing still, COP is directly below the COG, and ground reaction force is the same magnitude as gravity but in the opposite direction. Gravity and ground reaction forces are on the same action line and cancel each other.

This basic relationship between COP and COG is maintained as long as the human body is stationary even if posture changes. In other words, COP is directly below the COG.

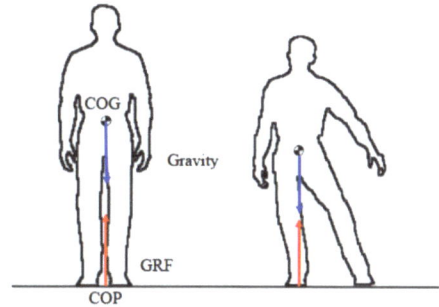

Base of support

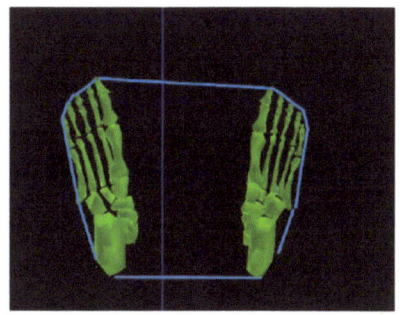

The outline formed around the feet in contact with the floor, as illustrated in the figure, is called the base of support. If the projection point of the center of gravity projected onto the floor, is inside the base of the support, the object can remain stable. When determining the base of support, please draw a figure of the feet that is in contact with the floor and encircle the figure with a large rubber band. The inside of the rubber band is the base of support. In theory, the COP can exist anywhere within this base of support. Conversely, the range in which COP can exist is the base of the support.

Center of Pressure (COP)

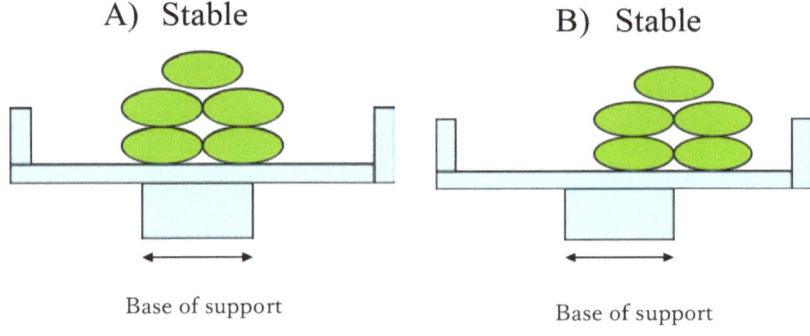

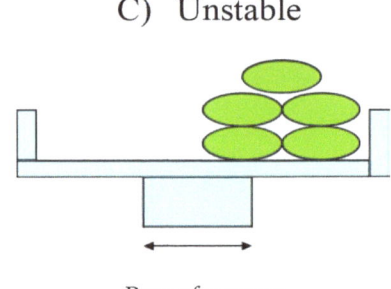

Let's consider why there is stability when the COG is within the base of support. There are donuts on a plate with a leg as shown in the example above.

In Figure A, the COG is inside the base of the support, so the donuts do not fall.

In Figure B, the COG is at the edge of the base of the support, but the donuts do not fall.

In Figure C, the COG deviates outside the base of the support, so the donuts fall. This is because the COP cannot extend outside the base to catch the COG.

Center of Gravity and Center of Pressure

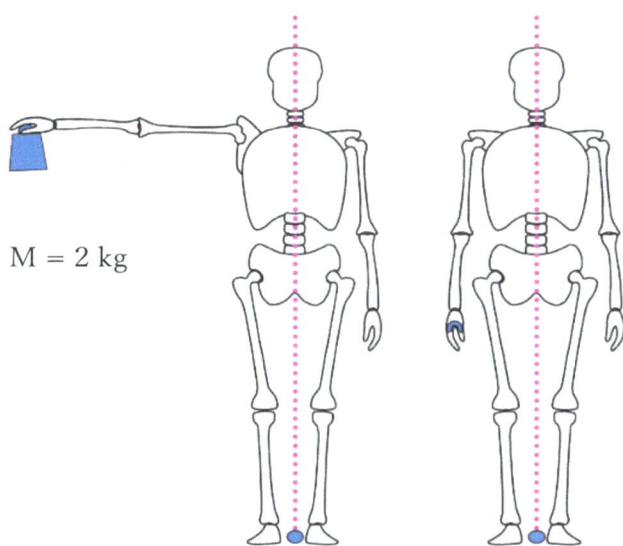

Let's apply it after mastering the basic principle. How will your posture change when you are standing and holding a mass of 2 kg with your right hand as shown in the figure? At this time, how will the COG and COP change?

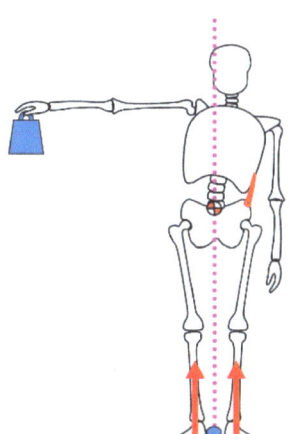

Let's think about it using two methods. The first method is to change posture. The upper body tilts in the opposite direction to balance the mass. The COP position does not change. The ground reaction force of the left and right feet remains the same. A certain amount of muscle activity is required to tilt the upper body. However, since the mass and the upper body's gravity are balanced, the thoracic region does not require much muscle activity. Nevertheless, the right shoulder must have a large abductor strength.

The second method does not change the apparent posture. Although the apparent posture is not changed, the position of the COP changes because of the combined center of gravity of the object mass and the body. Therefore, the ground reaction force of the foot with the object mass increases and the opposite side decreases. Also, considering the spinal column as the center, the center of gravity of the upper part shifts toward the object mass to balance the lever system. Increased muscular activity is necessary in the thorax. As in this example, if you look at it for a while, it may appear that less muscle activity is required if you do not change your posture. One of the purposes of learning biomechanics is to be able to understand that these illusions may be wrong.

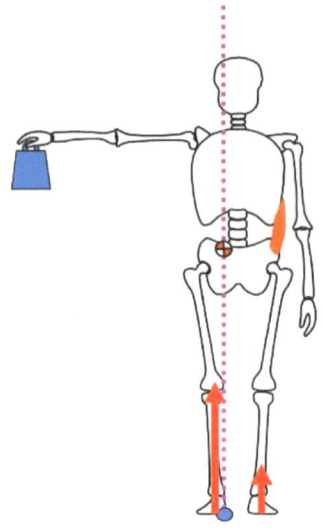

Even in this case, this posture cannot be maintained if the combined center of gravity deviates from the base of the support plane.

Therefore, there is a limit to the object mass that can be lifted in this position.

Reach movement

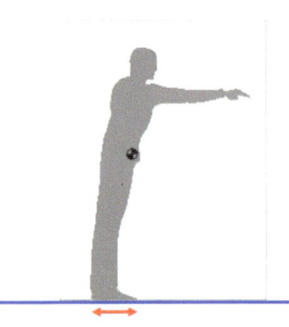

Base of support

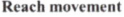

Let's think about reaching out to a position with your hand extended in front. In this case, the center of gravity moves slightly forward as much as the hand and the body lean forward. You can move the center of gravity up to the front edge of the base of support, but if you move it further forward, you will fall.

Now let's consider the sitting position.

The basics are the same for the sitting position. The center of gravity must be within the base of support consisting of the foot and the seating surface.

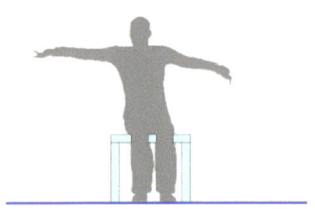

Fundamental Biomechanics

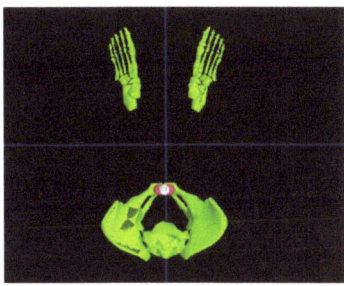 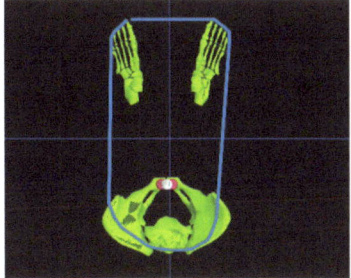

Try to draw the base of the support in the seated position. Draw an illustration of the sitting posture from above, and draw the base of the support on it.

For teachers
The chair base is not related to the base of the support. The drawing is based on the contact surface of the feet and the contact surface of the buttocks.

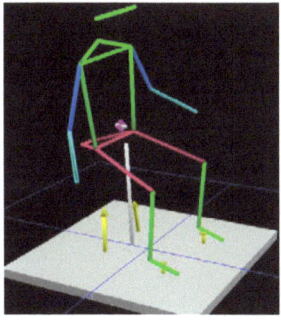 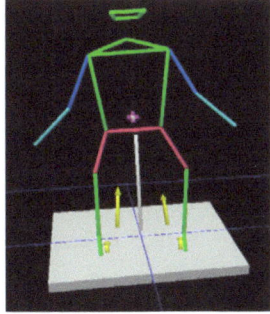

Note that in the relaxed sitting position, the ground reaction force, which is a combination of the ground reaction force of the feet and buttocks, is oriented vertically and is located directly below the COG.

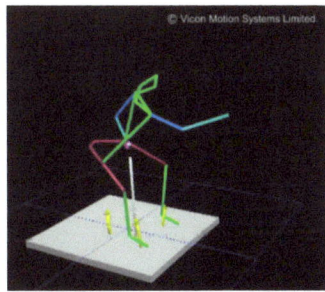

An example of forward reaching. This person loads a lot on the right leg when sticking out his right hand. In other words, the COG moves to the right front. Correspondingly, the floor reaction force action point, or COP, also move to the right. Overall, the load on the buttocks has decreased and the load on the feet has increased. The ground reaction forces on

Center of Pressure (COP)

the buttocks and feet tilted from the vertical, but the tilting forces cancel each other. You can see that the combined ground reaction force is vertical.

This is an example of reaching to the right side. The COG moves to the right, and correspondingly, most of the load is applied to the right buttock. Again, the COP is located directly below the COG. Note that the ground reaction force applied to the buttocks and feet are in the opposite direction, and the combined ground reaction force is vertical.

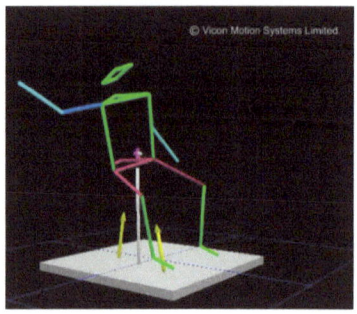

SUMMARY
- The range where the COP can move is the base of the support.
- At the stationary position, there is stability if the COP is directly under the COG.

CHAPTER 7

Joint Moments and Muscular Activities

On completion of this chapter, you will be able:

1. To explain joint moments
2. To tell how to calculate the joint moments
3. To explain the relationship between joint moments and ground reaction forces

The Joint moment is one of the essential concepts in biomechanics because joint moments are closely related to muscle activity. The common term "muscle strength" is used in daily life. It most likely refers to the joint moment.

Joint Moments

Before considering muscular activities, it is necessary to think about the balance of moments of force. Let's review the balance of the lever system. If a mass is placed on the right side of the lever in the figure, gravity corresponding to the mass will occur. This force causes a moment of force to rotate the lever clockwise. A mass is necessary on the left side of the center of rotation to make the lever system standstill. Because of this mass on the left side, a counterclockwise of the moment of force occurs, so that the lever system can become stationary. The balanced equation of the moment of force at this time is as follows:

$$F1 \times h1 = F2 \times h2.$$

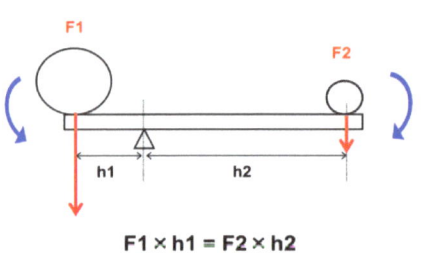

$F1 \times h1 = F2 \times h2$

When considering the lever system in the human body, the center of rotation is the center of the joint, the force from one mass is the external force, and the other is the muscle strength.

Let's consider the external forces applied to the body. First, let's consider muscle activities in the upper limbs. Consider the case when the elbow flexor muscle activity is measured while pulling the spring scale at a distance from the elbow joint, as shown in the figure. Assume that the elbow does not flex or extend because the moments of the flexor muscle and the spring are balanced. In this state, the moment of the force that the spring tries to extend the elbow is expressed as the value of the spring force **F1** multiplied by the distance **a** from the center of the elbow joint to the force action line. The balanced moments of muscular force cause the flexor muscle to flex the elbow. The value is obtained by multiplying the force **F2** of the elbow flexor muscle by the distance **b** from the elbow joint perpendicular to the line of action of **F2**. Therefore, the balance equation between the two moments is as follows:

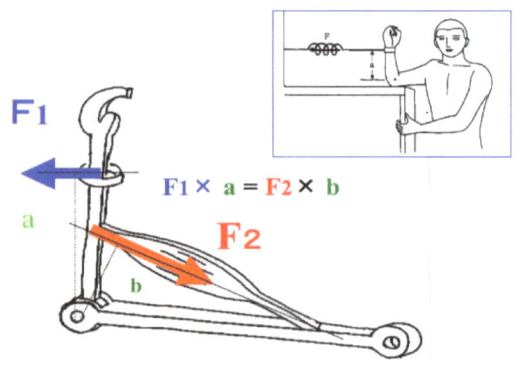

$F1 \times a = F2 \times b$

F1 × a = F2 × b.

At this time, the action of muscle tension rotating the joint, **F2 × b** is called the joint moment. The joint moment can be accurately determined if the external force **F1** and the distance **a** are known. In this way, the joint moment can be calculated by knowing the moment of the external force. Since **F1** is a force, the unit is **N** (Newton), and **a** is a length, so the unit is **meter**. Therefore, the unit of the joint moment is **Nm** (Newton meter). The joint moment increases when the external force **F1** is larger and when the distance **a** from the rotation center to the force action line is larger.

Muscle torque

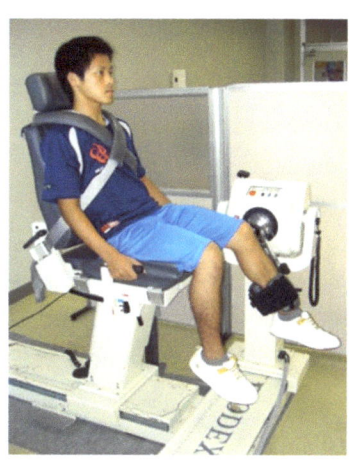

Now let's consider the case of the lower limbs. The figure shows a measuring instrument that measures muscle "strength". This machine measures the moment of the knee extensor muscle by externally applying a load to the knee with a motor. The value measured by this machine is also called knee torque in the sports field. The moment of force and the torque are almost the same concept in this context. Therefore, the unit of muscle torque is also Nm (Newton meter).

We can measure muscle "strength" by using this machine. However, if we want to know the muscle "strength" generated during daily life, what can we do? We cannot use this machine in these contexts.

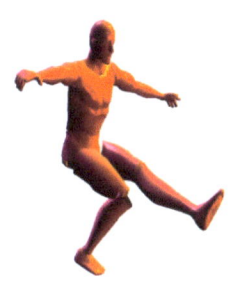

Consider standing on one leg and bending your knee, as shown in the figure. Knee extensor muscle activity is necessary. What is the external load to the knee for this posture? If you have a substantial bodyweight, the load is likely heavy. When you move your body up and down quickly, the external load will be large. In other words, the weight of the body above the knee joint and the way the body moves will influence the load on the knee joint. Therefore, if the weight and movement of the body above the knee joint are accurately measured, the joint moments of the knee joint can be obtained. However, since it is difficult to measure this accurately, we will consider the force applied below the knee joint. The greatest external force acting on the part below the knee joint is the ground reaction force. As we have studied so far, the ground reaction force reflects the bodyweight and the movement of the center of gravity. The joint moment of the lower limb can be obtained by considering the ground reaction force.

Joint Moments and Ground Reaction Force

First, let's consider the force applied to the foot when a human is standing. The ground reaction force acts on the foot from the floor upward. Assume the ankle joint is the center of rotation of the lever system. The ground reaction force is the force acting upward from the right side of the center of rotation.

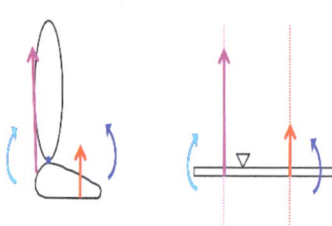

This force causes the lever to receive a counterclockwise moment of force. An upward force is required on the opposite side of the center of rotation to counter this. In the case of the foot, the force of the plantar flexor muscles acts, creating a clockwise moment of force, and the lever balances. To maintain a particular posture in this way, the muscle on the opposite side of the ground reaction force vector works around the joint (center of rotation). The moment of ground reaction force and muscle strength are not perfectly balanced. However, it is reasonable to assume that the two are almost balanced in a slow movement such as daily movement.

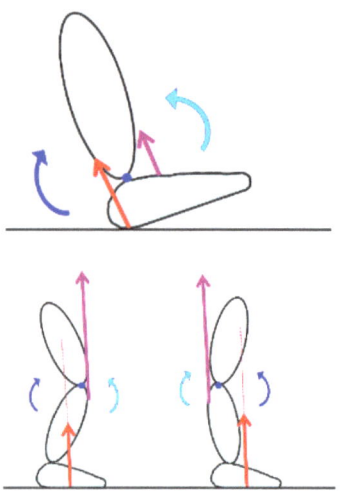

As shown in the figure, when the ground reaction force acts on the heel, the action line of the GRF vector passes behind the ankle joint, so the dorsiflexor works to counter this.

When thinking about the knee joint, for the sake of simplicity, the lower leg and foot are considered as one segment. Think about how the ground reaction force moves the segment. Then, as observed with the ankle joint, if the action line of the ground reaction force vector passes behind the knee joint, the knee extensor muscles work to counter this. If it passes in front of the knee, you can see that the knee flexor muscles work.

The Magnitude of the Joint Moments

Next, let's consider the magnitude of the joint moment. Suppose there is a mass near the fulcrum.

Even if the mass is the same, the moment of force applied to the lever increases as the distance from the fulcrum becomes larger.

The same is true for joint moments. Consider the situation when the COP moves from the middle of the foot to the toes area.

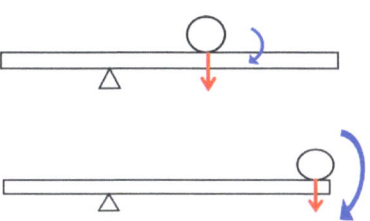

The farther the force vector is from the center of rotation, the larger the magnitude of the moment of force.

To maintain a posture with the COP on the toes, a larger activity of the plantar flexor muscle is necessary. This increment is because the COP moved forward. It may be easier to understand that the COP has moved forward due to increased muscle activity. In this way, even if the ground reaction force is the same size, a larger joint moment is required if it acts far from the joint.

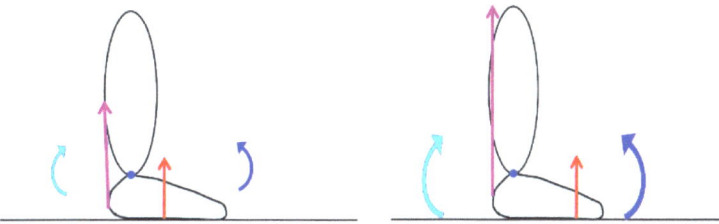

📝 For teachers

Please make all students stand up on the spot. With eyes closed and relaxed in a natural anatomical position. Let them imagine that the center of gravity of the body is in the center of the pelvis. At the same time, let them imagine that the COP is directly below the center of gravity. The position of the COP is around the middle of the foot and in front of the ankle joint. From this state, slowly move the center of gravity forward, and with that, the COP will move just below the center of gravity. Please be aware that the activity of the triceps surae muscle will increase at this time. Next, slowly move the center of gravity backward to be directly above the ankle joint. At this time, let them recognize that the activity of the triceps surae muscle reduces.

Joint moments during Knee Flexed Posture

Let's consider whole-body movement. Consider a posture where the knees are bent, and the trunk is tilted forward. Let's observe the relationship between the ground reaction force and lower limb joint moments. The action line of the ground reaction force vector passes in front of the ankle joint, behind the knee joint, and in front of the hip joint. As a result, the ground reaction force causes the ankle joint to dorsiflex, the knee joint to flex, and the hip joint to flex.

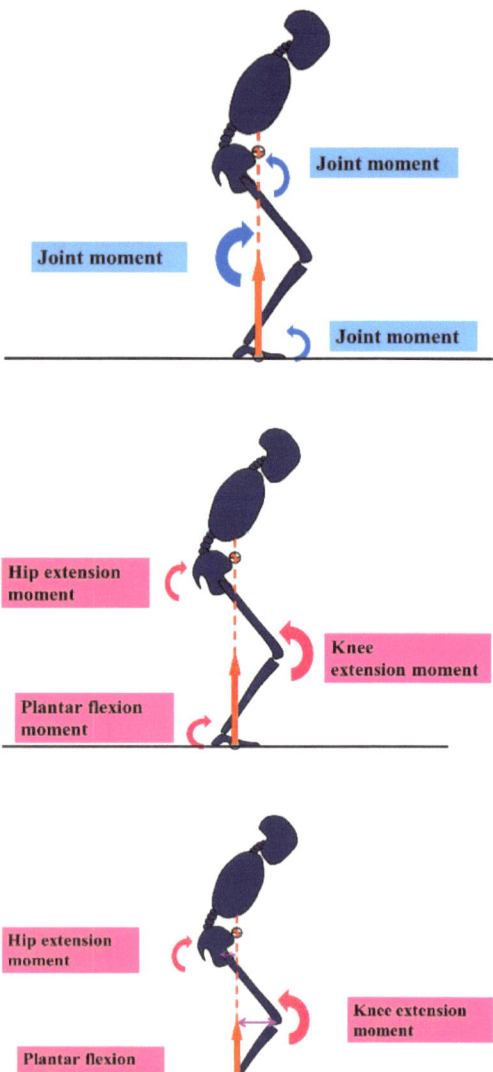

The joint moments at this time are in the opposite direction of the ground reaction moment around each joint. In other words, plantarflexion moment, knee extension moment, and hip extension moment are considered to be active.

The magnitude of the joint moments is determined by the distance from each joint to the ground reaction force vector. In this figure, since the distance from the knee joint to the ground reaction force vector is large, the extension moment of the knee joint is large.

Fundamental Biomechanics

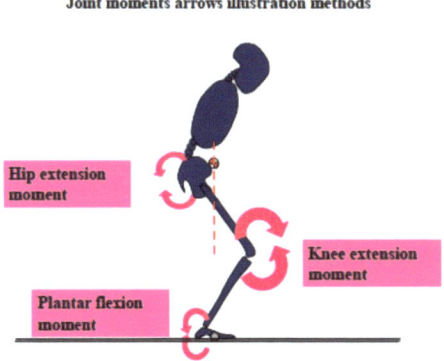

Joint moments arrows illustration methods

Now let's learn a new technique on how to draw joint moment arrows. There is always an origin and insertion for the muscle. One segment usually has the muscle origin at the distal end and the adjacent segment usually has the muscle insertion at the proximal end. When the muscles are shortened, both segments rotate and approach each other with the joint as the axis of rotation. Draw two pairs of joint moment arrows as shown in the figure to get an image of such an action. Make sure that the tips of both arrows face each other in the center. With this drawing method, you can always imagine the normal effects of joint moments. It can be recalled that, for example, the hip extension moment has the effect of pulling the knee backwards and at the same time pulling the trunk backwards when the hips are extended. It can be seen that the extension moment of the knee joint has the effect of making both the thigh and lower leg perpendicular to the ground in the posture shown in the figure, and the plantar flexion moment of the ankle joint firmly holds the forefoot. At the same time as pressing it against the ground, you can imagine that it has the effect of helping to raise the lower leg vertically.

If squatting is further increased, the distance from each joint to the ground reaction force vector increases. The joint moments increase as well for each joint. Let's illustrate the joint moment at this time with the new technique that we have just learned. Please get used to this drawing method as soon as possible.

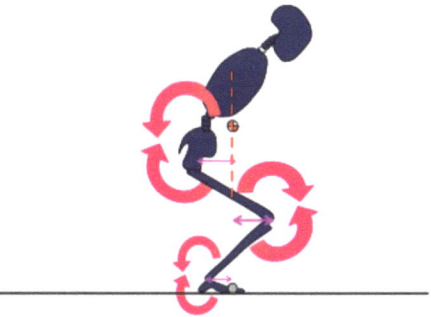

Joint moment with knee flexion

Joint Moments and Muscular Activities

For teachers

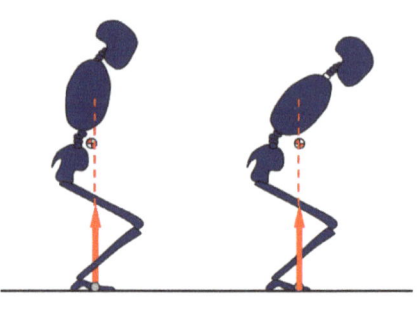

Please let the student stand in the natural anatomical posture and let them imagine the position of the center of gravity. Next, let them imagine the position of the COP for each of the right and left feet. Please keep the upper body upright and bend the knee joints to about 90° so that the activity of the knee extension muscles will increase. At this time, they can feel that the left and right ground reaction forces pass considerably behind the knee joints. From this posture, ask them to slowly tilt the trunk forward, and let them feel the center of gravity move ahead. They can observe that the ground reaction force on the left and right gradually move forward. One can feel that the knee extension muscles become less active as the ground reaction force comes nearer to the knee.

SUMMARY
The amount of joint moment required for each joint varies depending on how far the ground reaction force passes from the joint.

📎 For teachers
Explain the contents of this reference section only if there are questions from students.

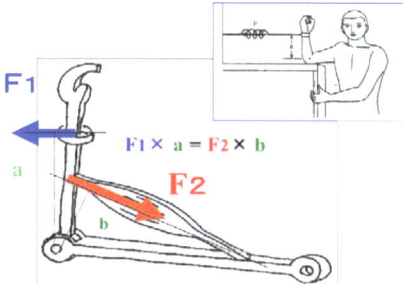

Calculation of the Upper Limb Joint Moment

When considering the joint moment of the upper limb, it is fundamental to calculate from the external forces applied to the upper limb, as shown in the figure. To calculate more accurately, consider the weight of the hand and forearm. If the balance is not perfect, consider the forearm movement (inertial force). If no external force is applied, only the weight and inertial force should be considered. When calculating the joint moment of the upper limb in this way, calculate the elbow joint moment by using the force applied to the hand. Use it to calculate the shoulder joint moments if necessary.

In the model in the figure, the trunk extension moment is related to the moment to extend the thigh as "action/reaction". Therefore, the hip joint moment in the posture shown in the figure can be calculated by the gravity applied to the part above the hip joint. In this case, consider gravity applied to the center of gravity of the trunk + head + upper limbs above the hip joint.

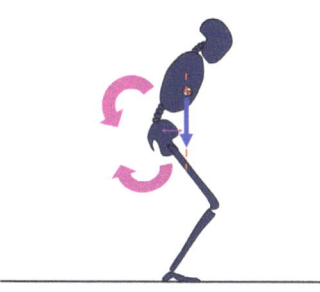

The value obtained by multiplying this gravity by the distance from the gravity action line to the hip joint is the trunk extension moment. The more you tilt your trunk, the larger the trunk moment becomes. If you have a heavy object in your hand in this posture, you will need a larger trunk extension moment as well. In this way, calculate from the top to calculate the moments of the upper limbs and trunk.

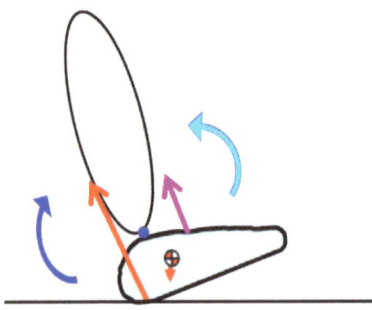

Calculation of the Ankle Joint Moment

In the case of the lower limb, the calculation starts from the bottom, that is, from the foot. The external force acting on the foot is the ground reaction force. In this figure, to be precise, the gravity and inertial force applied to the foot's center of gravity must be taken into account. However, since the ground reaction force is very large compared to gravity and the inertial force, even considering only the action of the ground reaction force, the joint moment can be estimated almost certainly.

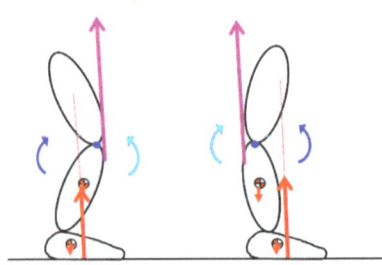

Calculation of the Knee Joint Moment

In the case of knee joints, it is necessary to consider the gravity and inertial force of the lower leg and foot. Gravity is always downward, and the direction is opposite to the upward ground reaction force. Therefore, the moment due to gravity works in the opposite direction to the moment of the ground reaction force. In this way, the joint moment will be different from the value when considering only the ground reaction force. However, since the influence of the ground reaction force is greater, there is not much difference.

Similarly, when considering the hip joint, the gravity and inertial force of the thigh, the shank, and the foot should be considered. As they are proximal joints, elements other than the ground reaction force increase. The difference between the joint moment considered only by the ground reaction force and the actual joint moment is largest in the hip joint. Of course, the effects of gravity and inertial forces are taken into account in the calculated joint moment. In this way, we calculate the joint moment of the lower limbs from the bottom. In other words, the joint moment is determined by considering the force applied to the distal (peripheral) side of the target joint in both the upper and lower limbs.

CHAPTER 8

Joint Power

On completion of this chapter, you will be able:

1. To explain the meaning of joint power
2. To explain mechanical work
3. To explain the work generated by muscles
4. To explain the power generated by muscles
5. To explain the relationship between power and muscle contraction

The term "power" is used in everyday life, such as "that person has power". However, we use it without knowing what it means. In biomechanics, this term must be used correctly. High power means not only great strength but also a quick movement is necessary. Let's understand the power correctly.

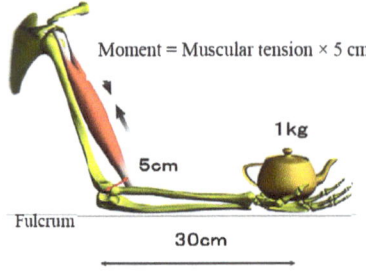

In the previous example illustrated in the figure, the joint moment of elbow flexion is 5 cm multiplied by the biceps muscle tension.

Mechanical Work

Before proceeding, let's review some physics. Suppose that you move the object on the floor with force as shown in the figure.

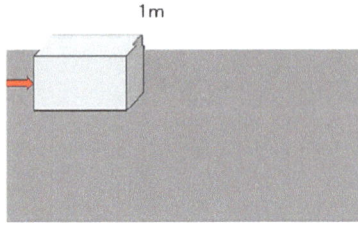

"force × distance" is called mechanical work. The unit of work is J (Joules).

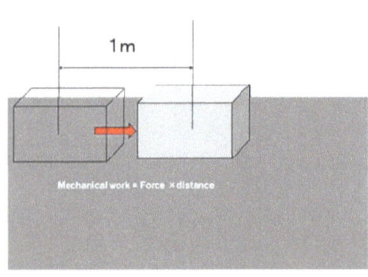

The value obtained by dividing this mechanical work by the time taken to move the object is called the work rate, or work per unit time.

Therefore "work = force × traveled distance", and
"work rate = (force × traveled distance) / time".

In the second half of the work rate formula, the traveled distance divided by the time is the velocity, so this equation can also be written as, "work rate = force × velocity".

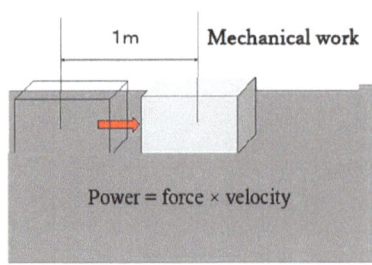

The work rate is called power. The unit is W (Watt). For this reason, the power increases when the force and velocity become larger.

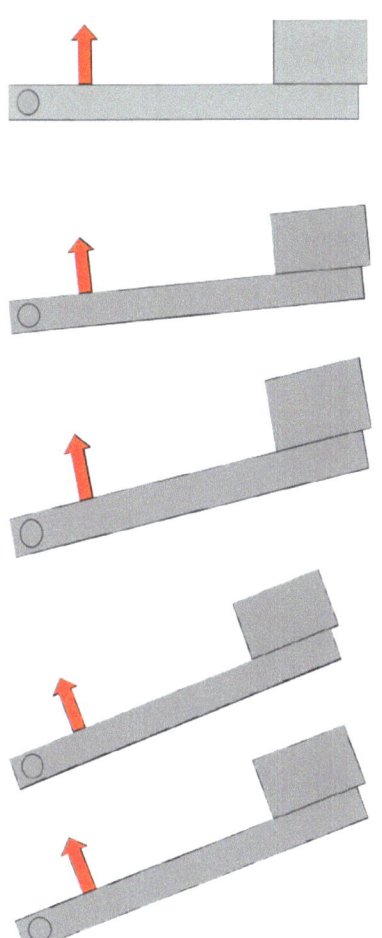

Muscular Activity and Work Rate

Now let's apply this idea in vivo. If you draw a model of lifting a teapot with your biceps, it will look like this figure. The left edge of this figure is the elbow joint. The red arrow represents the biceps muscular force. For simplicity, the biceps force is represented perpendicularly to the forearm.

When the biceps contract, the forearm rotates as shown in the figure, and the teapot goes up.

> At this time, pay attention to the biceps tension and the movement of the insertion point.

Joint Power

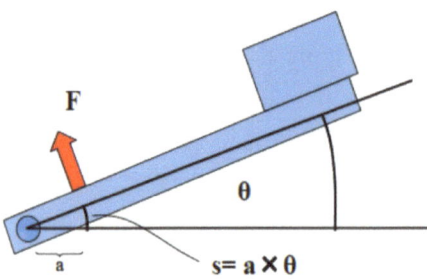

Work = F × s = F × a × θ = M × θ

Rotation movement

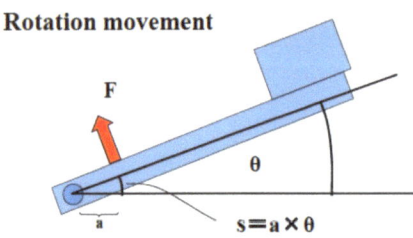

Work = F × s = F × a × θ = M × θ
Work rate = Work/time = M × θ/time
= M × Angular velocity

The distance where the insertion of the biceps has moved is **s** in the figure. The **s** is an arc of a circle with radius **a**. This value is expressed in mathematics as "**a** × θ". θ is the angle in radian.

The work of the biceps is **F** × **s**, so rewriting **s** with "**a** × θ" will result in "work = **F** × **a** × θ".

"**F** × **a**" in the first half of this equation is the joint moment.

That is, "work = joint moment × θ".

The work rate (power) is the work value divided by time. Dividing θ by time results in the angular velocity. Therefore, the power of the biceps is "joint moment × angular velocity". The power increases when both the joint moment and angular velocity become larger.

Joint Moments and Muscular Activities

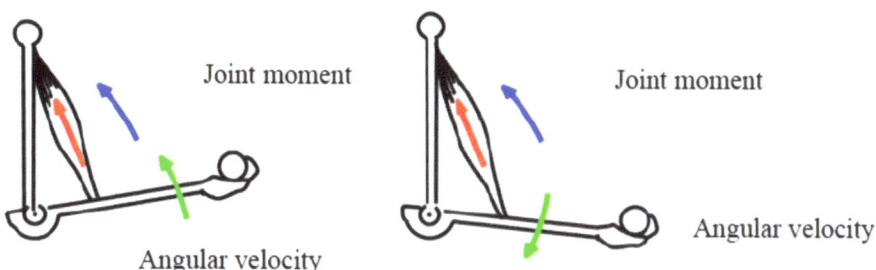

Positive power   **Negative power**

By knowing the joint moment and the angular velocity during movement, it is possible to estimate the state of the muscle contraction. Let's consider the case where the elbow is flexed, as shown in the figure. At this time, the flexor muscles are activated and generate an elbow flexion moment. When flexing the elbow joint from this state, it will bend while generating a flexion moment. It can be said that the elbow flexor has a concentric contraction.

On the other hand, when extending the elbow joint from the posture shown in the figure, it will extend while generating a flexion moment. The elbow flexor muscles have an eccentric contraction. The gravity extends the elbow joint while the joint moment decelerates the movement.

Power around the Joint

Power = joint moment × joint angular velocity
Positive power: concentric contraction or shortening contraction
Negative power: eccentric contraction or extensible contraction

By calculating the power around the joint from the results of motion analysis, you can quantitatively investigate the function of such muscles. Joint power can be calculated from the calculated joint moment and angular velocity. The mathematical definition of power is the joint moment multiplied by the angular velocity of the joint. The power is equivalent to the work that the joint moment does in a unit time. If the direction of the joint moment and the direction of angular velocity are the same, the power is positive, corresponding to concentric contraction. When the joint moment and the angular velocity directions are opposite to each other, the power is negative and corresponds to eccentric contraction. If a muscle generates a moment without changing the joint angle, it can be said that the muscle is isometrically contracted. In this case, the angle does not change, so the angular velocity is zero, and the power becomes zero.

Types of Muscle Activity

There are three different forms of muscle contractions.
Isometric contraction: Muscle length does not change
Concentric contraction: Joint moment and joint movement are in the same direction
Eccentric contraction: Joint moment and joint movement are in the opposite direction

Muscle activity can be divided into three categories according to changes in muscle length during activity. Isometric contraction generates force without changing its muscle length. Concentric contraction generates force while shortening the length of the muscle. Eccentric contraction generates force while the length of the muscle stretches. Considering muscle activity during movement, concentric contraction is when the knee extends while the knee extension muscles work. That is when the joint moment and joint movement have the same direction. Conversely, eccentric contraction is when the knee flexes while the knee extension muscles work. That is when the joint moment and joint movement are in the opposite direction.

Since concentric contraction is when the muscles generate positive work, in the case of a robot, energy is required to activate the electric motor. Since eccentric contraction is when the muscles generate negative work, in the case of a robot, energy is not required because the muscle acts as rubber or a spring. However, even in this case, the muscles of humans consume metabolic energy.

Muscles Activities during Squatting

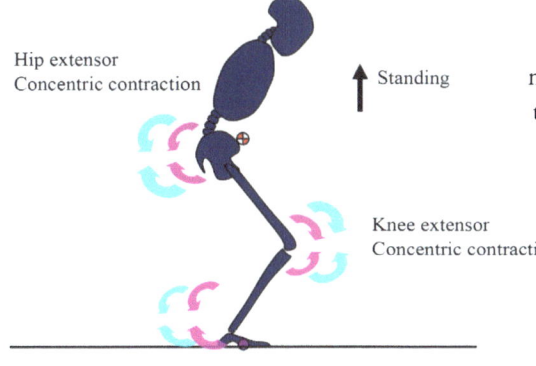

This figure shows standing movement. In this state, the ankle plantar flexor, knee extensor, and hip extensor muscles are active. At the start of the movement, the ankle joint is plantarflexed, while the knee and hip joints are extended. The joint moments and the movement of the joint are in the same direction. The muscle activity for all three joints, in this case, is a concentric contraction. If you calculate the power, all three joints' power will be positive. In this state, muscle activity overcomes the ground reaction force and lifts the center of gravity upward.

Muscles Activities during Squatting

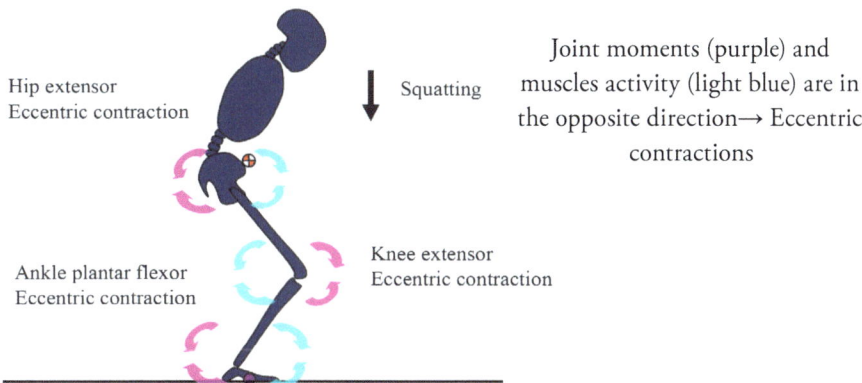

This figure shows a squatting movement. The muscles that are active around each joint are the same as standing movement, but the joint movements are ankle dorsiflexion, knee flexion, and hip flexion. Muscle activity is eccentric contraction because the joint moments and joint movements are in opposite directions. If you calculate the power, all three joints will be a negative power. The falling movement is generated by gravity. The falling movement by gravity is braked (decelerated) by the muscles around each joint. It should be noted that the working muscles are both extensor muscles when raising and lowering the body. When rising, it will be easy to imagine that the extensor is working. But it might be difficult to imagine that the extensor is working when lowering the body. In this case, it is gravity that causes the joint to flex, and the muscle groups are braking to do this slowly and smoothly.

In the standing position, the lower limbs are always pushed by the ground reaction force. In order to maintain the body posture in this state, activities of extensor and plantar flexor muscles are necessary. These muscles are therefore called antigravity muscles.

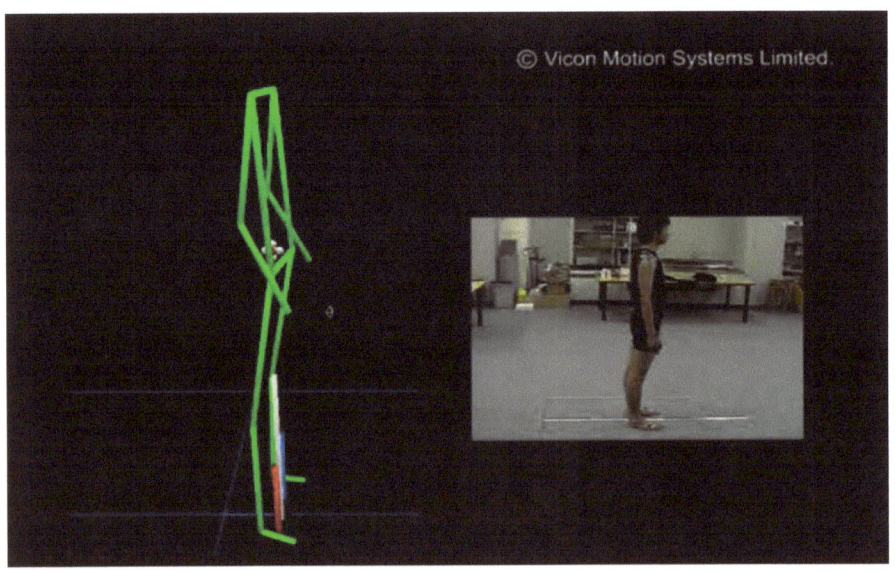

For teachers
You can repeat the squatting computer graphic polygons and let the students imagine the joint moments and joint movements.

Synergistic and Antagonistic Muscles Joint Moments

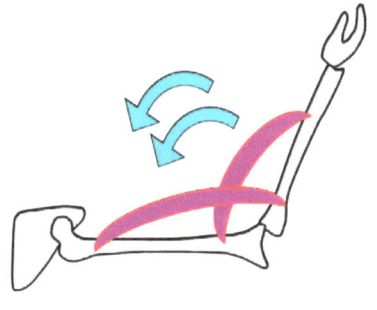 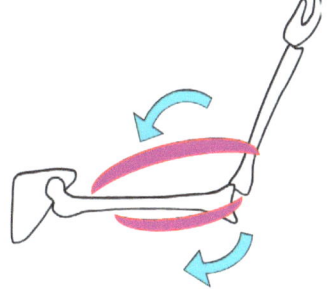

Joint moment
(Sum of synergistic muscles)

Joint moment
(Difference between synergistic and antagonistic muscles)

Here we explain the limitations of the concept of joint moments. The joint moment is the sum of the moments of force inside the body. The force inside the body is not only muscle force. For example, it includes forces generated by tissues such as ligaments and joint capsules around joints. Furthermore, even if only muscle force is considered, synergistic and antagonistic muscles are acting as shown in the figure. The joint moment is the sum of the moments generated by these forces. In the case of synergistic muscles, it is the sum of these moments. In the case of antagonistic muscles, the joint moment is the difference between the moment of these muscles. The activity of individual muscles cannot be determined from the results of joint moments alone. It is necessary to measure the electromyogram (EMG) to know the muscular activity of each muscle during movement.

Joint Moments and EMG Comparison

Finally, let's compare the joint moment and EMG. Since joint moments can be expressed quantitatively in Nm units, comparison between individuals is easy. On the other hand, the electromyogram displays a percentage of the maximum muscle contraction, making it difficult to compare different people. In the joint moment, for example, the ankle joint flexor moment is expressed as the sum of the activities of the flexors. This can make it difficult to identify which muscle of the triceps surae is active. A surface electromyogram allows you to know individual muscle activities except for deep muscles. Thus, it is necessary to understand and utilize the characteristics of joint moments and electromyogram.

Comparison between Joint Moments measurement and EMG

	Joint moments	EMG
Quantitatively	Excellent	Fair
Individual Muscle Activity	Fair	Excellent

CHAPTER 9

Jump Movement

On completion of this chapter, you will be able:

1. To explain mechanical energy
2. To explain muscle activity and jump height
3. To explain ground reaction force and center of gravity acceleration during jumping
4. To explain the joint moments during jumping
5. To explain the power of joint moments during jumping
6. To explain how to jump high

We will use all of the knowledge we have learned so far to analyze a jump movement.

> **Mechanical Energy**
>
> Kinetic energy is "$K = (1/2) M \times V^2$"
> Potential energy is "$U = M \times g \times h$"
> where M: mass, V: velocity,
> g: gravitational acceleration, h: height

Mechanical Energy

First, essential knowledge regarding energy are as follows:

The Kinetic energy is "$K = (1/2) M \times V^2$"

The Potential energy is "$U = M \times g \times h$"

where M: mass, V: velocity,
g: gravitational acceleration, h: height

Assignment

How many meters will the center of gravity rise when a person weighing 65 kg jumps vertically upward at an initial velocity of 3.0 m / s?

Answer

The idea is that if the initial velocity is 3.0 m / s, the kinetic energy will be

"$K = (1/2) M \times (3.0 \text{ m/s})^2$".

At the highest point, kinetic energy is all converted to potential energy, so K becomes U,

"$U = K$"
"$M \times g \times h = (1/2) M \times (3.0 \text{ m/s})^2$".

> External force → acceleration
>
> Work → kinetic energy
>
> Muscles do mechanical work

When h (height) is calculated from this, h = 0.45 m.

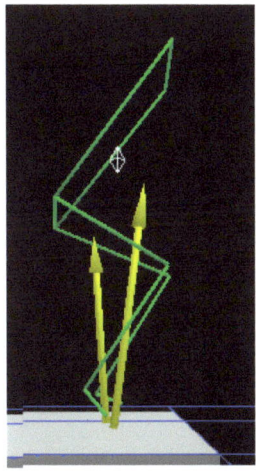

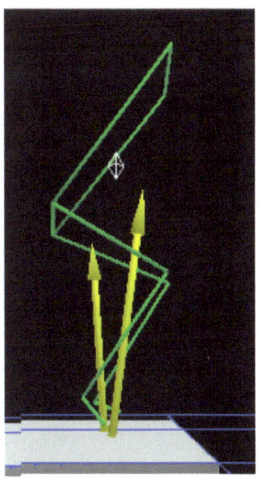

The following should be noted in the above assignment. The center of gravity was stationary at the beginning, and just when the foot was leaving the ground, the velocity of COG was 3.0 m / s. It means that the force was acting on the body while the foot was on the ground. Although this force is a ground reaction force, a large force that cannot be canceled by gravity is applied for the required time. The second point is that kinetic energy is generated at an initial velocity of 3.0 m / s. Something must have worked for energy to be created. It was the concentric contraction of the joints' extensor muscles that worked. In other words, the extensor muscle group showed positive power in the time zone before jumping up. Since power is a work per unit time, if power is used for a certain period, the accumulated amount becomes work. This work creates kinetic energy for jumping up. Pay close attention to these two points before proceeding to the next task.

Jump Biomechanics

First, observe the jumping movement in the PowerPoint. Next, draw a graph of the change in the height of the center of gravity during this movement.

Jump Movement

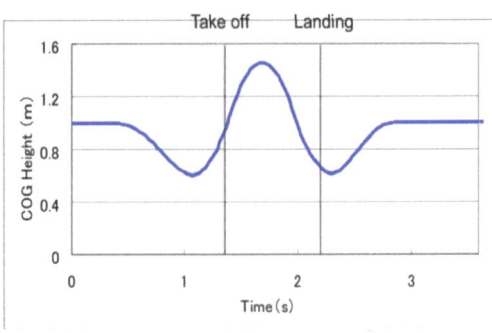

Graph of COG height during the jumping movement

📌 For teachers
Please draw a graph of the height of the center of gravity during jumping. The horizontal axis is time, and the vertical axis is the height of the center of gravity. Indicate the time of take-off and landing with vertical lines so that you can see the time zone when jumping from the ground.

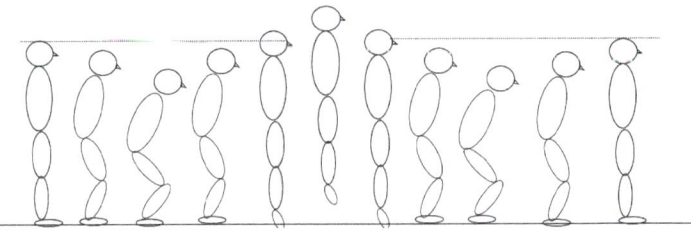

Let us consider the velocity of the center of gravity during the jump movement.

📌 For teachers
Let the students think about the center of gravity velocity, drawing the center of gravity height and the actual movement in mind. Consider the direction and magnitude of the velocity at each time point in the slide. The velocity is positive during upward movement and negative during downward movement. Ask all of the students to stand up and simulate the vertical jump movement in slow motion to understand the velocity change. At first, the velocity becomes negative from zero when squatting and from zero to positive during rising. The maximum velocity is positive at the time of takeoff. The velocity then becomes zero at the highest point of the center of gravity. Then at the moment of landing, the maximum velocity becomes negative. After that, the negative velocity once again becomes zero as the COG comes to the lowest position. When the COG rises, the velocity becomes positive and returns to zero.

While jumping, let us draw a graph of the ground reaction force for the first half of squatting and jumping.

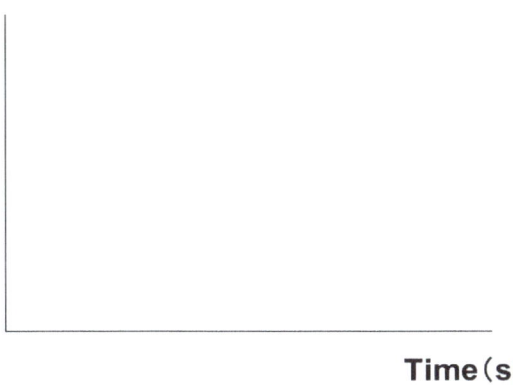

Time(s)

📓 **For teachers**

Next is the ground reaction force. Let the students draw a graph of the vertical component of the ground reaction force from resting to squatting. The ground reaction force becomes zero during jumping in the air. The horizontal axis is time, and the vertical axis is the vertical ground reaction force.

The vertical ground reaction force

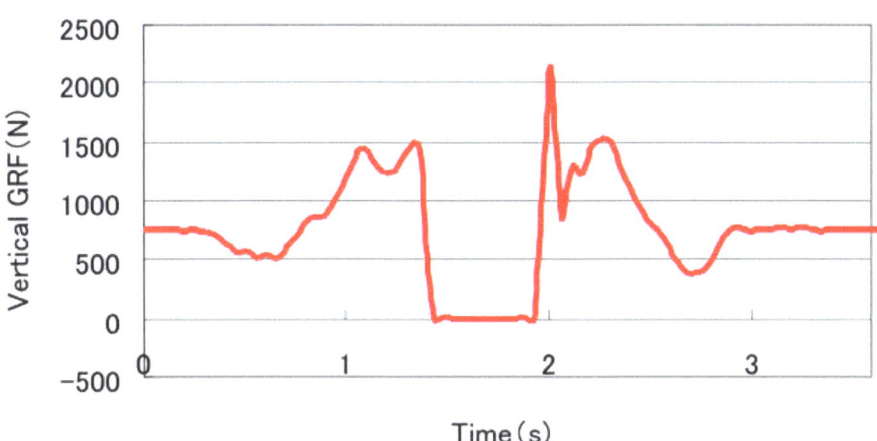

📓 **For teachers**

Present this graph after students draw the graph. Students draw the first half of this graph. The graph is the vertical component of the ground reaction force, including jumping up and landing. The ground reaction force, which has the same value as the gravitational force when standing still, initially becomes smaller than the gravitational force and then increases. The ground reaction force is zero when jumping in the air. A large ground reaction force acts at the moment of landing, and then it again gets smaller and then returns to its original value. Let the students understand that the ground reaction force first becomes smaller than the gravitational force before jumping and then becomes larger than the gravitational force. Let the students think about why the ground reaction force first becomes smaller than the gravitational force and then increases. Many students mistakenly understand that the ground reaction force returns to the gravitational force level at the lowest position of the center of gravity. Let the student stand and repeat knee flexion and extension, and to understand that a large ground reaction force returns at the lowest position of the center of gravity.

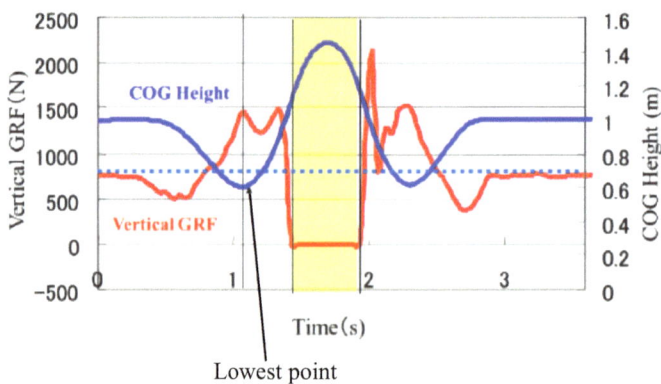

COG Height and Vertical Ground Reaction Force

Lowest point

Let us check this with a graph. This graph is drawn by overlaying the height of the center of gravity and the ground reaction force in the vertical direction. During the first half of squatting, the ground reaction force is below the gravitational force line. After crossing the gravitational force line in the second half of squatting, the ground reaction force reaches a peak before jumping up at the lowest height of the center of gravity.

COG vertical acceleration

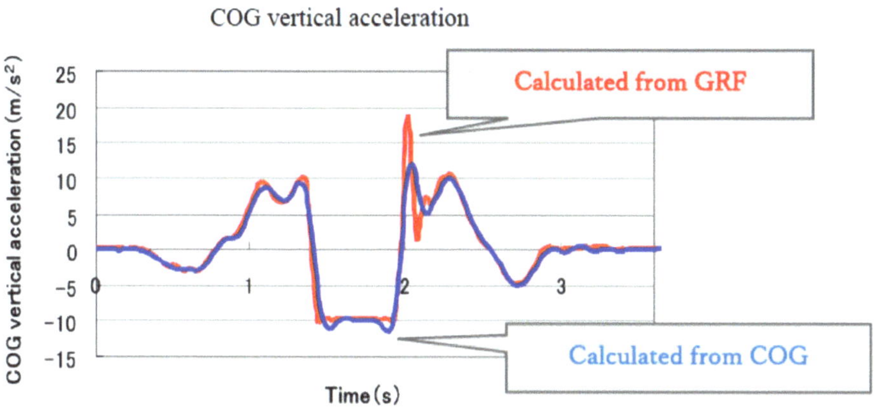

This graph compares the acceleration of the center of gravity calculated from the center of gravity and calculated from the ground reaction force. You can see that both are in good agreement. You observe that Newton's equation of motion can be applied to body movement.

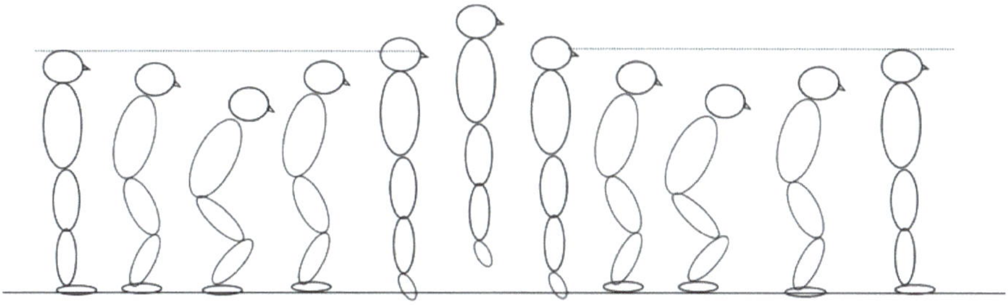

Next, let us think about knee joint movement and muscle activities during jumping.

For teachers

Let the students think about the movement and muscle activity of the knee joint by simulating a jumping movement.

Jump Movement

Assignment

Fill in the table below for knee joint movement and muscle activity during the jumping. The movement begins with Squatting and moves to Extension of the joints. The Jump occurs and then Squatting happens again to end with Extension of the joints.

	Squatting	Extension	Jump	Squatting	Extension
Joint motion (Flexion-Extension)					
Joint moment (Flexion-Extension)					
Contraction type					

For teachers

Make the students fill in the table above for knee joint movement and muscle activity during the jumping. Please show the jump movement repeatedly in the video while checking the ground reaction force vector and the knee joint position.

Answer

	Squatting	Extension	Jump	Squatting	Extension
Joint motion (Flexion-Extension)	flexion	extension		flexion	extension
Joint moment (Flexion-Extension)	extension	extension		extension	extension
Contraction type	eccentric	concentric		eccentric	concentric

For teachers

The extensor muscles are always active around the knee joint during the jump movement. At the beginning of squatting, the knee joint flexes while the knee extensors are decelerating the motion. At this time, the COG is lowering due to gravity. Eventually, concentric activity begins, and the knee joint extends and the COG goes up. The vertical velocity increases and the body leaves the floor. At the time of landing, the knee extension muscles undergo eccentric contraction to absorb the shock, and the knee joint bends. Later, concentric activity begins, and the knees extend to return to a standing posture.

Fundamental Biomechanics

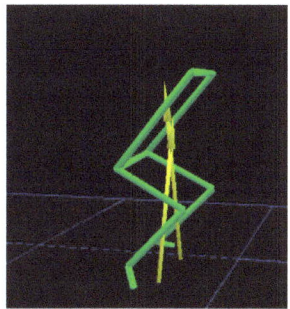

For teachers
While watching the PowerPoint, show that the trunk leans forward before jumping. Let the students think about the meaning of the trunk leaning forward. Let us think about the difference between a jump that does not tilt the trunk forward and a jump that does tilt the trunk forward. If you do not tilt your trunk forward, you will notice that you are not using the hip extension moment.

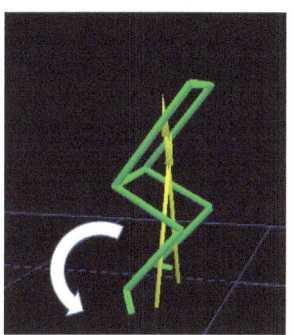

For teachers
Next, let us explain the action of the plantar flexor muscles in jumping. The plantar flexors work just before the body is thrown into the air. If the plantar flexor muscles are active from an early stage, the body moves backward rather than upward. Please let the students experience this.

Muscles used in the Jumping Movement (Hip extensor, Knee extensor, Ankle plantar flexor)

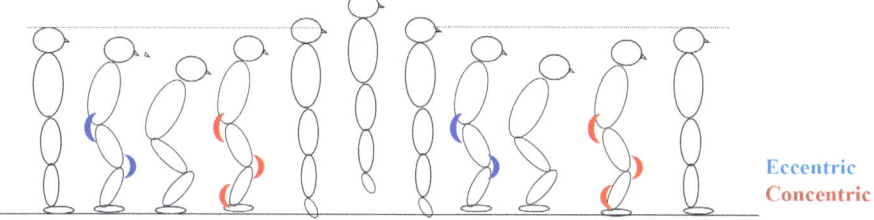

Eccentric
Concentric

SUMMARY

In summary, the extensor muscles are mainly active in all three joints. Initially, the three joints move in eccentric contraction during Squatting. The concentric contraction occurs in the extension movement phase. After landing the jump, the eccentric contraction occurs when Squatting. The concentric contraction occurs in the final extension phase. Overall, all the positive power generated by the muscles is absorbed by the muscles (negative power). Owing to the negative power, the muscles can minimize the impact on the body. If the muscles cannot absorb the shock, the bones, ligaments, and organs would absorb the shock, which can cause significant damage. In this way, the concentric contraction of the muscles before the jump generates a large positive power that throws the center of gravity into the air. Finally, let us observe the jumping motion again with a video while considering how the muscles work during the movements.

CHAPTER 10

Biomechanics while Rising from a Chair

On completion of this chapter, you will be able:

1. To explain the movement of the center of gravity while rising from a chair
2. To explain the meaning of the trunk tilting forward
3. To explain the change in the base of support and center of pressure
4. To explain changes in ground reaction force
5. To explain the activities of muscles while rising from a chair

During activities of daily living, we sit down on a chair and stand up from chair. However, if you learn biomechanics, you can observe how demanding the movement is. After understanding that, let us think about how to stand up easily using biomechanics.

Movement of the COG during standing up from a chair

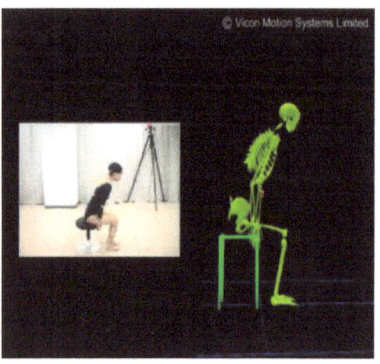

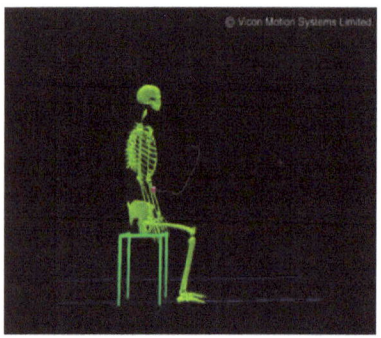

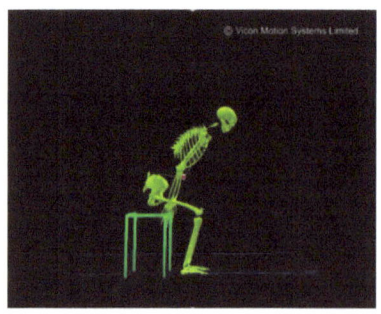

For teachers

Let four students perform the standing up movement from the chair. Which part of the body moved first? The head started to move first. From another perspective, the trunk started to move first rather than the head. In terms of motion analysis, the trunk first tilted forward. Why do you first tilt your trunk forward when you stand up?

Let us observe the video on the PowerPoint to think about this dynamically. The left half of the screen is a video. The right half is computer-graphic (CG). The white and red dots in the CG represent the calculated COG. When sitting, the COG is not in the middle of the pelvis, but near the navel. The COG that was near the navel, when you were sitting, will fit in the center of your pelvis at standing position. In this way, the COG is not always at a fixed position in the body. The position of the COG is determined by the mass distribution of the entire body. If the posture changes, the position of the COG will change.

To make it easier to understand the movement of the COG, the trajectory of the COG is shown. A trajectory is a trace that remains after an object moves like a contrail. If you draw the trajectory of the COG, you can see that the COG does not immediately go upward, but first moves forward. The COG does not just go forward but rather moves downward. Then, the COG changes the direction in the middle of the movement and goes upward.

Let us stop the computer graphic when the movement of the COG changes direction. What do you observe at this time? At this time, the buttocks are leaving the seat. Why?

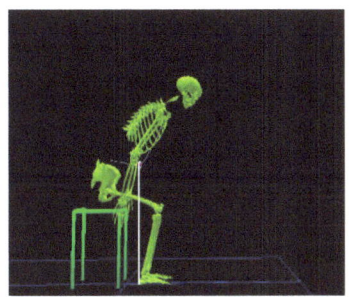

COG is in line with the end of the heel at the moment of buttocks leaving the seat

To think about this, let us draw a vertical line from the COG. Where does this vertical line pass? The vertical line from the COG passes just behind the heel. In other words, after the trunk tilted forward and the COG reached the edge of the heel, the buttocks left the seat.

Base of Support

Let us draw the base of support in the sitting position by looking at the sitting position from the top.

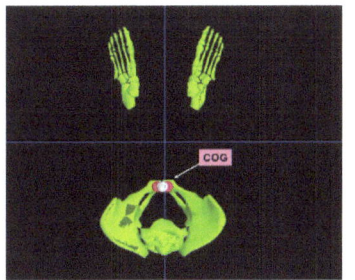

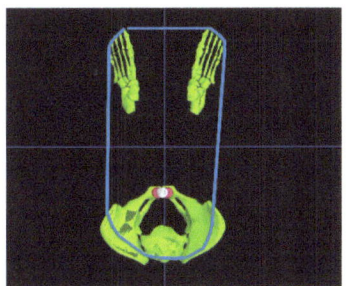

It looks like this when you look at the base of support from the top. The base of support consists of both feet and buttocks. When sitting, the center of gravity is in this base of support.

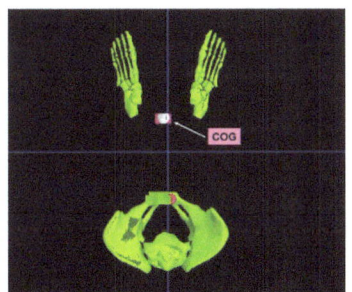

Next, let's draw the base of support when the buttocks leave the seat.

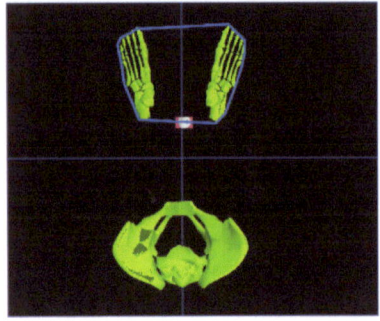

After the buttocks leave the seat, the base is only a narrow area made with both feet. If you move the buttocks away from the seat before the center of gravity enters the base of the support, the body will fall backwards. Therefore, we tilt the trunk forward and put the center of gravity into the base of the support made with both feet.

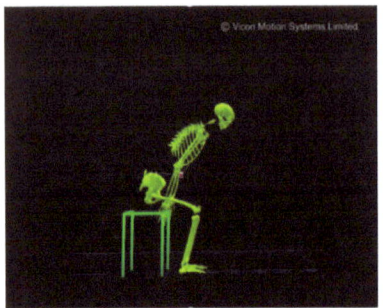

Meaning of the Trunk tilting forward
With this movement coordination in mind, let us take a look at the standing up video again. The COG needs to be in the foot sole when the buttocks leave the seat. You do not have to tilt your trunk as much when you put your feet near the buttocks beforehand. On the other hand, when you put the feet farther forward, the trunk must be tilted more forward when the buttocks leave the seat.

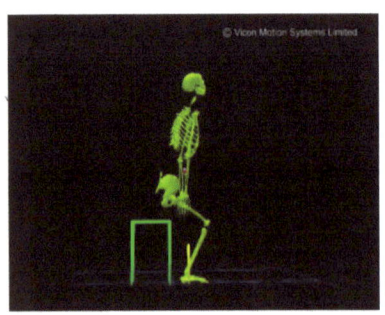

Next, let us observe standing up with the trunk upright as much as possible. What is the difference between typical standing up and standing with the trunk upright? It seems that the knee burden increases when standing with the trunk upright. Why is this so?

Muscle Activities during Standing up

In order to think about this, watch the video and CG of the normal way of standing up motion again. Let us pause the video at the time when the buttocks leave the seat. The burden on the knee becomes largest at this moment. Where does the ground reaction force pass? Pay attention to the relationship between the ground reaction force and the knee. Here, the action line of the ground reaction force vector is displayed as a white line. Also, pay close attention to the relationship between the white line and the knee joint. How far is the ground reaction force vector from the knee?

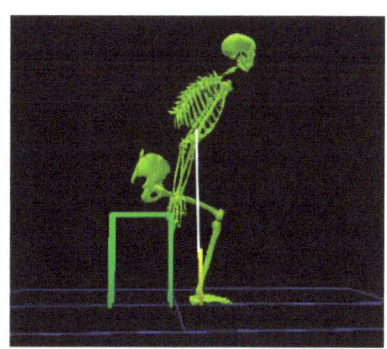

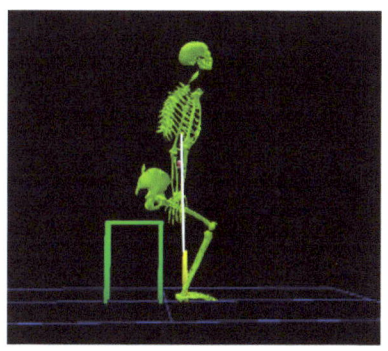

Next, let us observe when the trunk is upright. How far is the line of action of the ground reaction force when the buttocks leave the seat? Compared to the previous example, you can see that the ground reaction force vector passes more behind the knee. As learned in Chapter 7 about joint moments, when the ground reaction force moves away from the joint, the joint moment of that joint becomes larger. In other words, when the trunk is upright, the COG remains behind the knee. Then, the ground reaction force is also located behind the knee, so the line of action of the ground reaction force passes behind the knee. If the trunk is not tilted forward in this way, a larger knee extension moment is required. In addition, are there any joints that become less burdened when the trunk is upright? Please try it yourself.

Biomechanics while Rising from a Chair

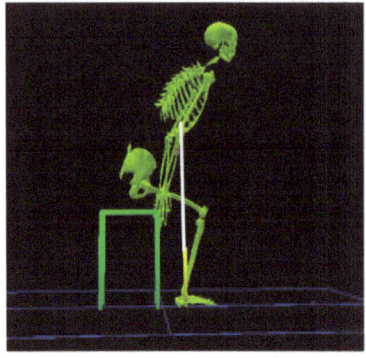 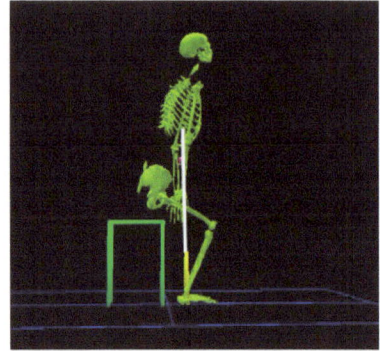

It turns out that the burden on the knee increases if the trunk is not tilted forward. Do you notice that the hip joint is not used at the same time?

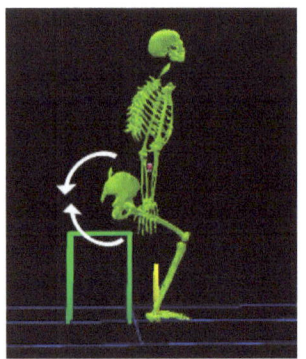

In other words, if the trunk is not tilted forward, the hip extension moment will be difficult to achieve. What happens if the hip extension moment is exerted without tilting forward?

📝 For teachers

From the seated position, let the hip extension muscles work while not tilting the trunk forward, and experience what happens. The trunk will rotate backward.

When the hip joint moment is exerted, the reaction causes a backward tilting moment to act on the trunk at the same time. Therefore, it is necessary to tilt the trunk in advance to apply a moment of backward tilt to the trunk safely. In other words, if the trunk is tilted forward, the hip extension moment can be used, and the knee extension moment can be reduced accordingly.

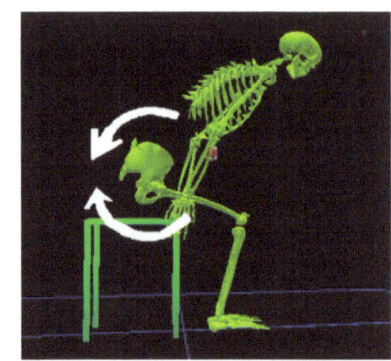

GRF of Standing up

Next, let us focus on the relationship between the ground reaction force and the movement of the COG. To make this easier to understand, here is a video of standing up quickly. Here, the ground reaction forces of the buttocks and feet are shown in yellow. The combined force of these is shown in white. The reaction force of the buttocks is the force acting on the buttocks from the seating surface, but here it is displayed as the force from the floor. The force vector can be moved along the line of action, so it does not matter if you display it either way.

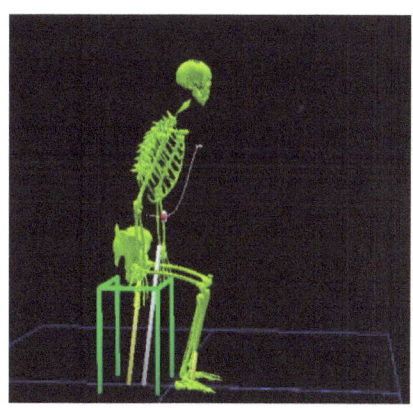

First, let us focus on the beginning of the movement. Do you notice anything when you start moving? You can see that the COP of the combined force moved slightly backward to go behind the center of gravity. The ground reaction force tilted forward to push the center of gravity forward. It looks like it is pushing the COG forward from the back.

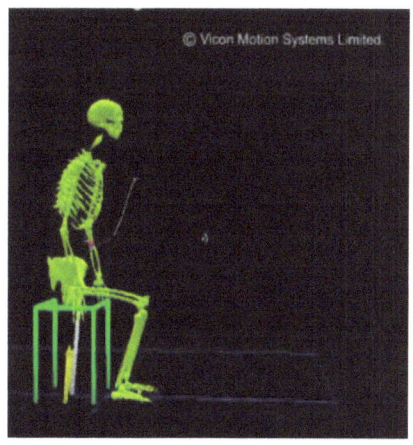

The video is played only during the beginning of the movement repeatedly so that you can observe the movement well. Why is the COP going backward at this time? The action of the hip flexor tilts the trunk forward slightly. As soon as the trunk leans forward, the moment of gravitational force acts on the trunk. If you lean forward a little, you can lean forward without doing anything.

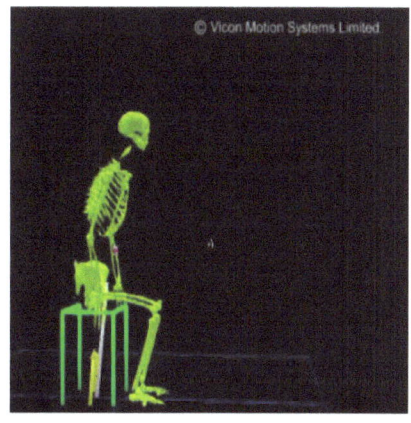

When the hip flexor is first activated, it will rotate the thigh. So, the knee tends to go up due to the thigh rotation. It is not really lifted. The moment is applied in the direction of raising the knee joint, reducing the load on the feet. As a result, the load applied to the sitting surface increases, and the force on the buttocks becomes dominant. The COP will move toward the buttocks area. This is the reason why the COP moves backward.

The COP is like a fulcrum that supports the whole body. When it moves backward from under the COG, the moment of gravitational force appears. The COG begins to rotate forward with the COP as a fulcrum. This rotation is reflected in the ground reaction force, and the ground reaction force tilts forward.

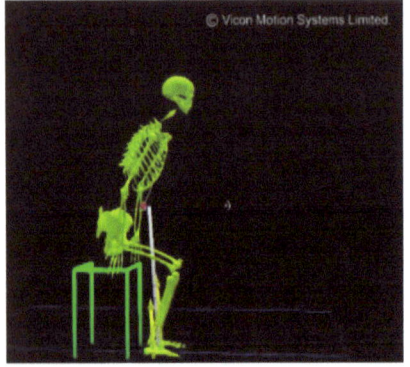

After this, the COP moves forward, and overtakes just below the center of gravity, and enters the base of support of the foot sole. After that, the ground reaction force tilts backward, decelerates the movement of the center of gravity, and moves the center of gravity upward.

When the center of gravity changes upward, the knee extension moment and hip extension moment reach their maximums, and the knee and hip joints extend. When extended, the ground reaction force passes closer to the knee and hip joints, and the extension moment of both joints becomes smaller. The knee and hip joints are coordinated so that the center of gravity remains above the narrow base of support. The COG moves smoothly upward without meandering, and the upright posture

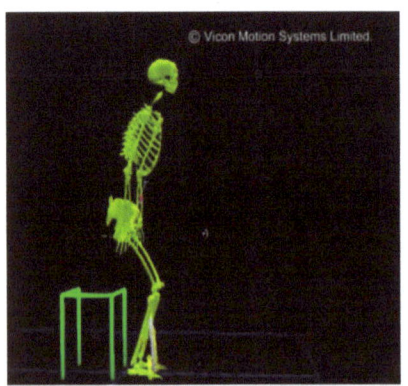

is completed. While the center of gravity moves upward, the ground reaction force vector is almost vertical, and the COP remains near the front of the ankle joint. It is the action of the ankle plantarflexion moment that keeps the COP in this position. In other words, during standing up, the ankle joint stabilizes the body by placing the rising COG above the base of support.

Fundamental Biomechanics

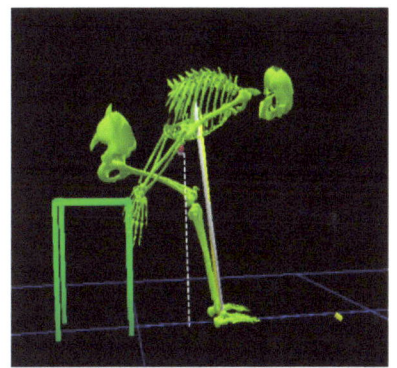

Watch the video and CG when you are sitting with your feet set more forward than usual. If you stand up quickly with sufficient momentum, you can lift the buttocks away from the seat before the COG enters the base of support of the feet. At the time of getting up off the buttocks, the COG is pulled back by the moment of gravitational force, but because there is momentum, it can escape into the base of support. However, this is not the case when you stand up slowly. If you do not put the center of gravity in the base of support of the feet, you will fall backwards. Therefore, it is necessary to lean forward in order to stand up slowly and safely. This leaning increases the burden on the hip joint.

Let us consider the occasion again when you are sitting with your feet more forward than usual. When the buttocks leave the seat, the dorsiflexor muscles are working, and the COP is located at the edge of the heel (the base of support limit). Also, at this point, the ground reaction force tilts backward, and the forward momentum is decelerated to convert it to upward movement. This is

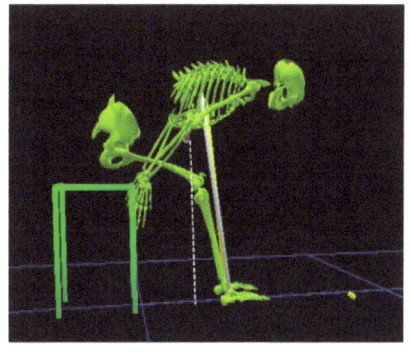

an extreme example, but even for the normal standing up, you will stand up easier if you are conscious of bringing the COP to the heel by activating your dorsiflexor muscles.

Case of using Handrails

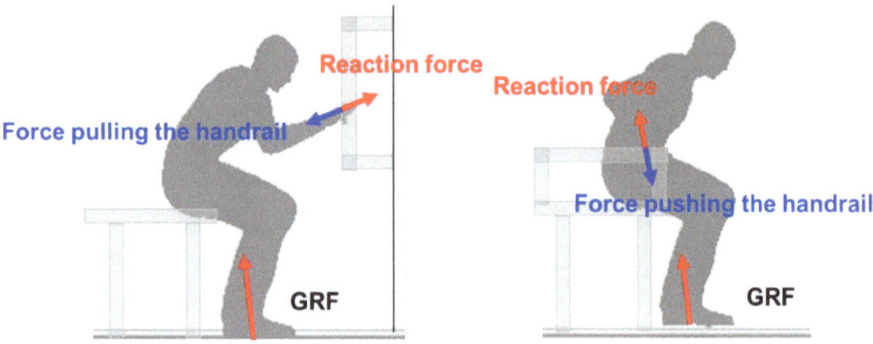

There are two ways to lighten the burden on the lower limbs when standing up. The first method is to bring the ground reaction force vector closer to the most active joint. The other method is to reduce the ground reaction force of the lower limbs with a handrail. When pulling handrails as shown on the left, the forward force from the handrails helps to move the trunk forward. When pushing on handrails as shown on the right, the upward force from the handrails reduces the ground reaction force on the lower limbs. It is important to focus on the reaction force that acts on the person from the handrail, not the force by which the person pulls or pushes the handrail.

CHAPTER 11

Biomechanics of Gait Initiation

On completion of this chapter, you will be able:

1. To explain the relationship between the center of gravity and COP when standing upright
2. To explain the movement of COP in sagittal and frontal planes during gait initiation
3. To explain the relationship between the movement of COG and COP
4. To explain the relationship between COP movement and joint moment
5. To explain the driving force to move the COG forward

Let's analyze the state of human walking dynamically. I think you will be surprised that the COP moves strangely.

Biomechanics of Gait Initiation

COG and COP during Standing

📋 For teachers

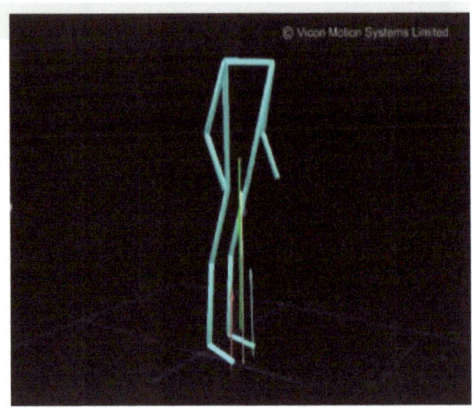

In this chapter, please explain to students by showing the computer graphic. The red arrow below the right foot is the ground reaction force vector of the right foot, the blue arrow is the ground reaction force vector of the left foot, and the white arrow is the combined left and right ground reaction force vector. The COP is at the base of each ground reaction force vector. In the computer graphic, the center of gravity (COG) is intentionally moving back and forth so that you can see the movement of the COP. You can see that the right and left COPs and the combined COP are aligned in a straight line. If the load on the right is large,

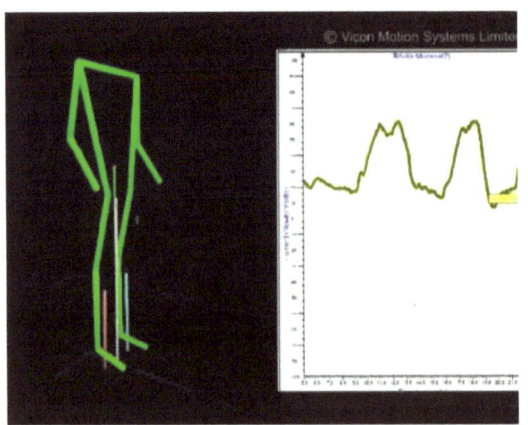

the COP will move to the right. If the load on the left is large, the COP will move to the left. You can see that the combined COP moves between the toes and just below the ankle.

During this movement, the ankle joint moment was calculated. The plantarflexion moment is positive and the dorsiflexion moment is negative on the graph. Let us compare the movement of the COP and the change in the ankle moment. It can be seen that the plantarflexion moment is large when the COP is around the toe, and the plantarflexion moment is small when it is close to the ankle.

COP movement during the Gait Initiation

With this background knowledge in mind, let us take a look at the first computer graphic of the walk. If you look at the movement of the COG, you can see it is moving forward smoothly. Please pay attention to the movement of the combined left-right foot COP just before initiation of gait. It can be noticed that the COP has been moving backwards. Moreover, if you observe carefully, the COP is moving to the left rear. The left foot is the first swinging foot. The load has moved toward the swinging foot. Why is this happening? In order to clarify this, let us consider the anteroposterior direction and the left-right direction separately.

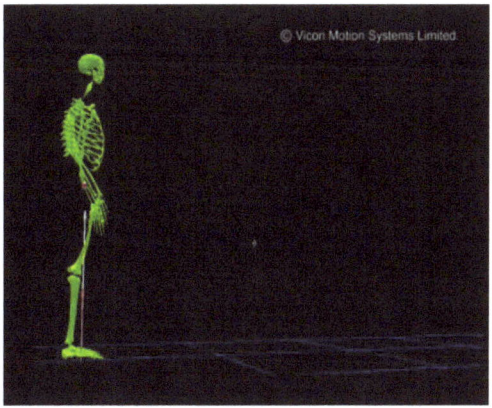

In the anteroposterior direction, let us think about the sagittal plane. Let us observe the time of the beginning of walking repeatedly. This time, we will focus on the ground reaction force of the right foot, which is the support leg, rather than the combined left-right reaction force. Indeed, the COP will first move backward. Recall the relationship between the COP and ankle plantarflexion moment when standing upright. Moving the COP backwards also means getting closer to the ankle joint. During that occasion, you can notice that the plantarflexion moment around the ankle joint is getting smaller. When the ankle plantarflexion moment is smaller, the COP moves from just below the COG to more posterior. Gravitational force always acts on the COG, and the moment of gravitational force appears when the COP is not just below

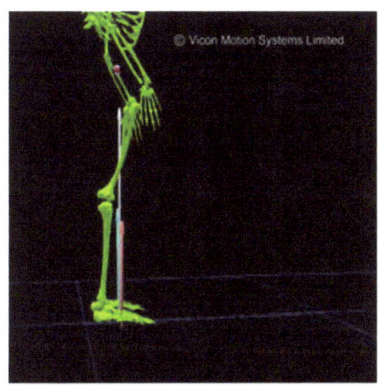

the COG. A COG which has lost support will fall forward. Correspondingly, the ground reaction force tilts forward. When the ground reaction force tilts, a horizontal component appears, which corresponds to the horizontal acceleration of the COG. In other words, the COP is moved backward to accelerate the COG forward. Please remember that the same phenomenon occurred when standing up from the chair (Chapter 10).

✏️ For teachers

Let the students stand and realize that the COP moves backward just before taking a step forward. It may be easier to understand if they move faster.

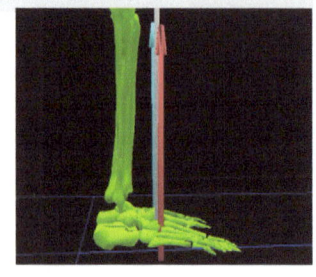

Now, let us observe the motion in the frontal plane from behind. Replay the computer graphic from the initiation of the gait to the time when the COP goes far to the left repeatedly. The first swinging foot is the left foot, but the COP has moved to the left of the swinging foot. Since the support point has moved to the left, the COG will move to the right. Due to the moment of gravitational force, the

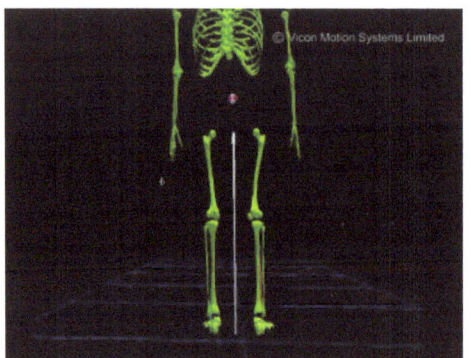

ground reaction force will tilt to the right accordingly. The situation is the same as the sagittal plane. How can this happen? Pay attention to the hip joint of the left foot. Do you notice that it is a little abducted? Also, pay attention to the hip joint of the right foot. Can you notice that it is a little adducted?

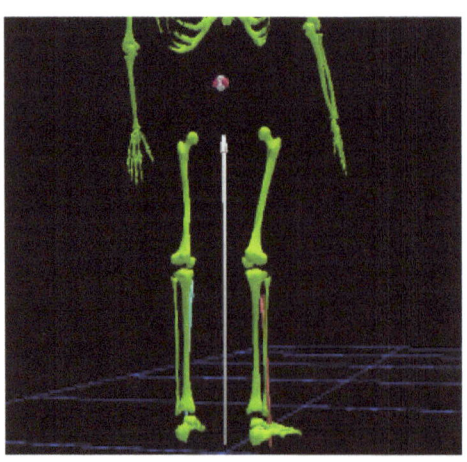

When the abductor muscle of the hip joint of the left leg is activated, the thigh is abducted. The reaction causes a moment that rotates the trunk to the left. Although it does not lead to side bending, this action reduces the load on the right foot. Pay attention to the ground reaction force of the right foot during this period. You can see that the right foot ground reaction force decreases for a while. If you strengthen the adductor of the hip joint of the right leg (or weaken the abductor), the thigh will adduct. The reaction causes a moment to rotate the trunk to the left, as seen from the posterior direction. Although it does not reach rotation, this action increases the load on the left foot. Pay attention to the ground reaction force of the left foot, which increases for a while. With changes in both of these ground reaction forces, the load on the swinging foot (left) foot increases and the load on supporting foot (right) decreases at the start of walking. This will cause the combined left-right COP to move to the left for a while.

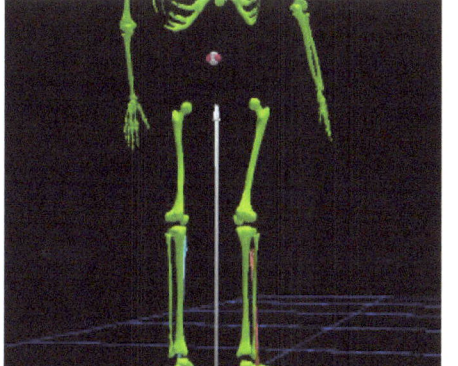

For teachers

Please let the students stand and spread their legs sideways within the width of the shoulders. While shifting the COG to the right foot, let students stand on one leg with the right foot. Make sure to feel that the COP moves temporarily to the opposite left leg.

Next, let us look at the computer graphic for the COG that moves according to the COP position.

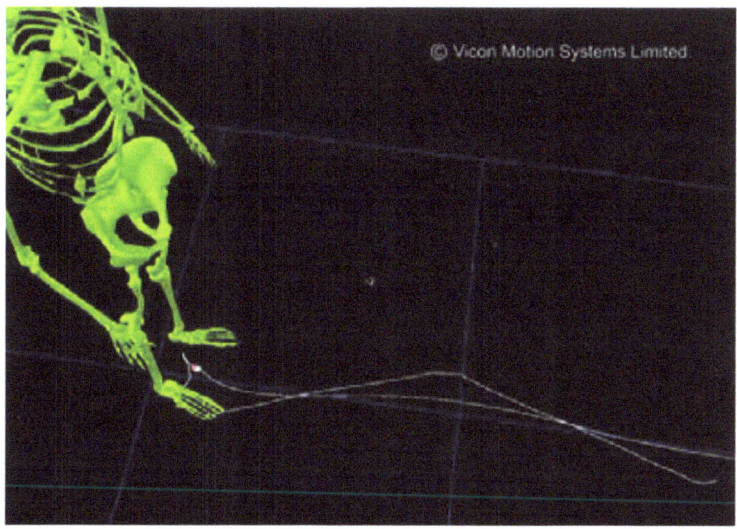

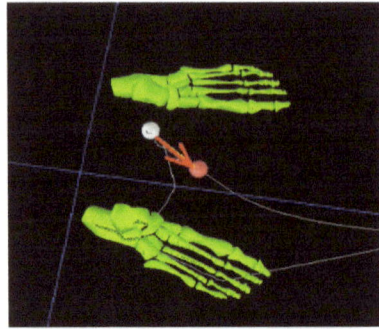

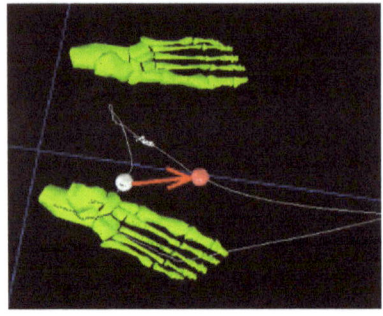

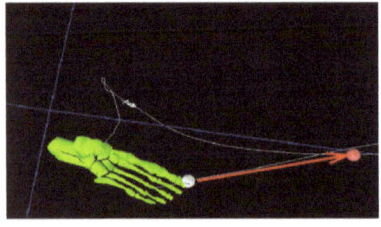

At the beginning of walking, we want to move the COG to the supporting leg (right leg) and forward. Then, the COP moves to the swinging leg (left leg). This results in a difference between the position of COP (white point) and the COG position projected on the floor (pink point). At this time, imagine that a force (red arrow) corresponding to the position difference acts from the COP toward the COG. Then, acceleration occurs in the direction of the force to the COG.

Let us move forward in time a little. At this time, a force acts from the COP toward the COG (this is an imagined force, and this red arrow does not become a force as it is drawn in the figure) and accelerates the COG. In this case, since the COG has already moved to the right and forward, the force acts diagonally from the side and the direction of COG is changed.

At this time, the gait initiation has advanced considerably. The COG is pushed out considerably from the back, so the COG is accelerated forward with a large acceleration. This is similar to the low pressure and high pressure changing the direction of a typhoon. Let us imagine that the COP adjusts the direction and velocity of the movement COG.

Fundamental Biomechanics

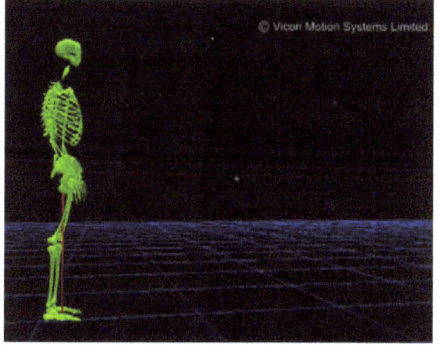

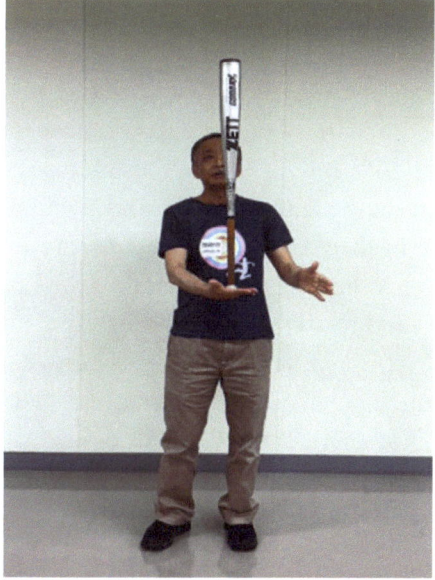

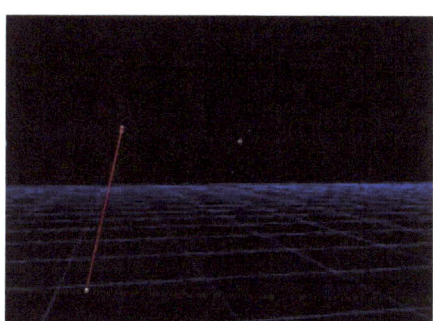

To emphasize the relationship between the COG and COP, the body has been removed from the computer graphic and a red line has been drawn to connect the COG to COP.

This is similar to keeping a standing baseball bat on the palm of your hand. In this activity, you must move your palm back and forth and left and right to keep the bat from falling. If you want to move the head of the bat forward, you should move your palm backward and push it forward with gravitational force. However, the bat will fall down as it is, so this time move your palm forward in front of the COG. Continue repeating the forward and backward movement of your palm, in order to keep the bat from falling. Please prepare a bat and try to move it back and forth while supporting it on your palm.

Let us emphasize again that the COP can be moved by relaxing the ankle plantar flexor muscles to move the COP backward. Or it can move laterally by changing the hip adductor and abductor moments. The COG cannot be moved directly. The COP can be moved by muscle activity, and acceleration of the COG occurs by changing the direction of the ground reaction force. The point is that the ground reaction force is changed according to the will of the person.

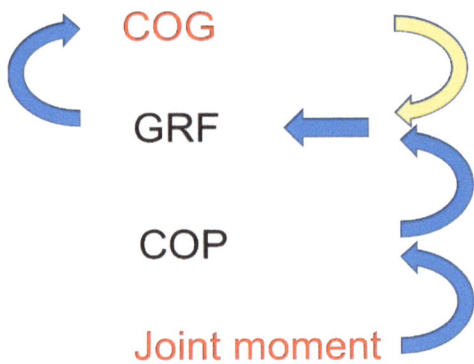

SUMMARY

The relationship of this concept can be summarized as shown in the figure. The joint moment changes the position of the center of pressure (COP). Due to the difference between the position of the COP and the COG, the anteroposterior direction and mediolateral direction components of the ground reaction force occur. The force causes acceleration in the COG, and the COG moves to determine the new position of the COG. When the position of the COG is determined, the anteroposterior direction and mediolateral direction components of the ground reaction forces are determined by the difference between that COG position and the COP position. The COG is further accelerated. This kind of chain reaction controls the movement of the COG as desired.

CHAPTER 12

Gait Biomechanics, Center of Gravity and Center of Pressure During Walking

On completion of this chapter, you will be able:

1. To explain the relationship between the center of gravity and center of pressure during walking
2. To explain the relationship between the center of pressure and joint moment during walking
3. To explain the relationship between the movement of the center of gravity and the ground reaction force

During gait initiation, we learned how the COP controls the center of gravity. Let us observe what happens in "normal steady gait" when the gait is stable and the velocity is almost constant.

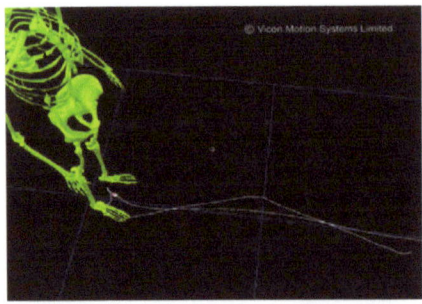

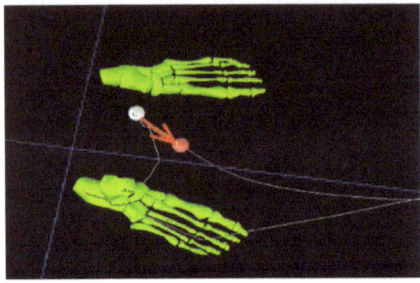

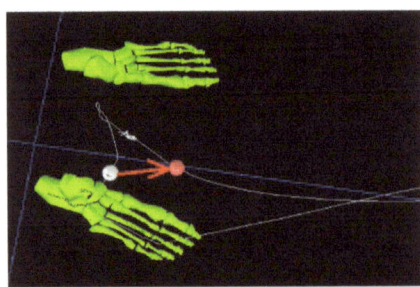

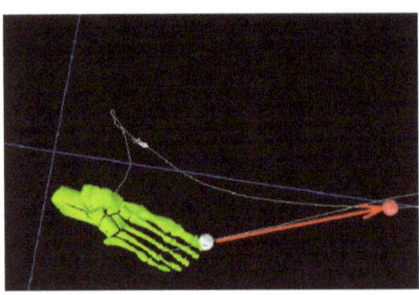

COG and COP during Gait

First, let us review the computer graphic of the COG according to the position of the COP at the beginning of walking.

At the beginning of walking, we want to move the COG to the right and forward, so we move the COP to the left and backward. This results in a difference between the position of COP (white point) and the COG position projected on the floor (pink point). At this time, imagine that a force (red arrow) corresponding to the position difference acts from the COP toward the COG. Then, acceleration occurs in the direction of the force at the COG.

Let us forward the time a little. At this time, a force acts from the COP toward the COG (this is an imagined force, and this red arrow does not become a force as it is drawn in the figure), causing the COG to accelerate. In this case, since the COG has already moved to the right and forward, the force acts diagonally from the side and the direction of COG is thus changed.

At this time, the gait initiation has advanced considerably. The COG is pushed out considerably from the back, so the COG is accelerated forward with a large acceleration. Once the gait initiation stage has completed (up until this 4th step), the walking will then remain constant.

Fundamental Biomechanics

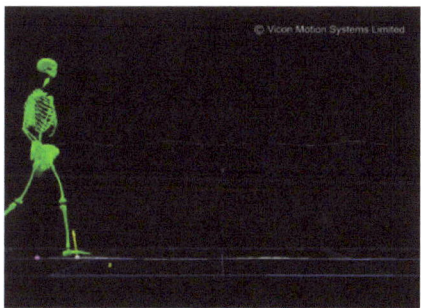

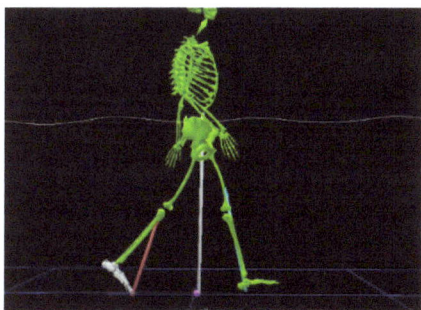

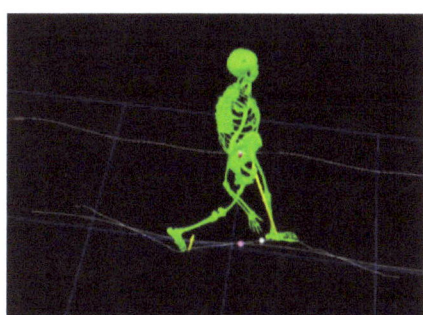

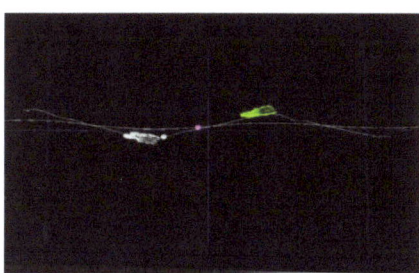

Let us use the computer graphic to observe the movement of the COG and the ground reaction force during walking.

Pay attention to the combined ground reaction force (white) of the left and right feet. The combined left and right COP position is determined by the balance between the load on the front foot and the load on the back foot. Therefore, the combined COP is behind the COG when only the back leg is in contact with the floor. When the front foot touches the floor, the COP begins to chase, catch up, and eventually overtake the COG at the position of the front foot. In this way, the combined COP controls the position of the COG by moving backward or forward in relation to the COG.

Looking from above, the COP does not only move to catch the COG in the forward and backward directions but also in the left and right directions. It looks as if the COP is handling the trajectory of the COG. The COP acts like a shepherd dog that moves the flock of sheep in the direction you want.

You can see this relationship clearly from the transverse plane.

Center of Gravity and the Base of Support

Let us apply the idea of the base of support here. In the two-leg support phase, the forefoot of the trailing (back) leg and the heel of the front leg contact the floor. The base of support is the area when we put the rubber band around the forefoot and heel in contact with the floor.

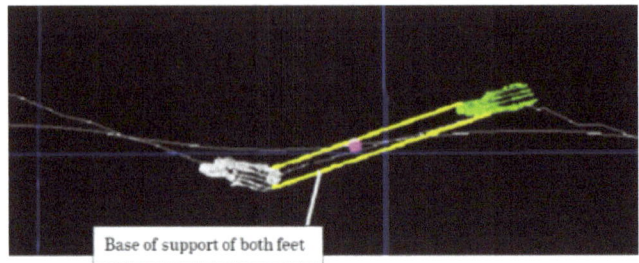

If you think about the base of support of one step before and after, a corridor becomes the base of support.

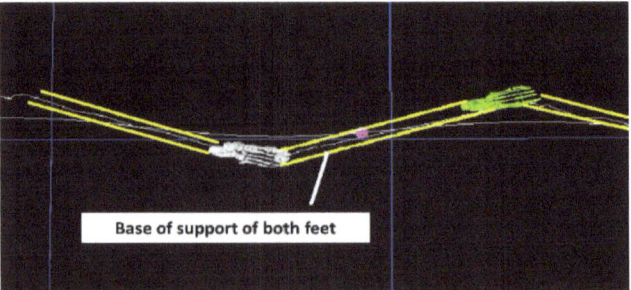

Since the footprint of the foot in the single-leg support period is the base of support, the narrow passage shown in the figure is the base of support, when connecting the base of all periods.

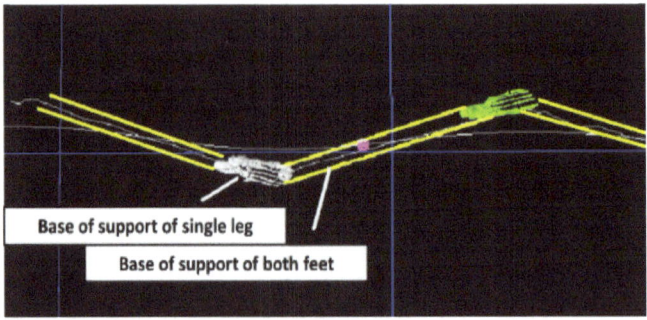

Keep in mind that the COG deviates from the base of support at all times during the single-leg support period.

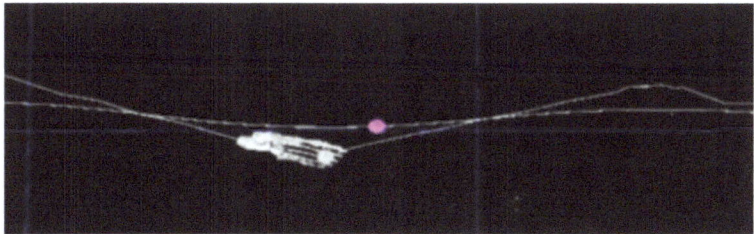

There is only a short time during the double support period when the COG enters the base of support. We can deduce here that regular walking is never a stable movement. Rather than being stable, it is more appropriate to describe walking as the COG moving forward while falling. So, in other words, an unstable state is continued smoothly and rhythmically.

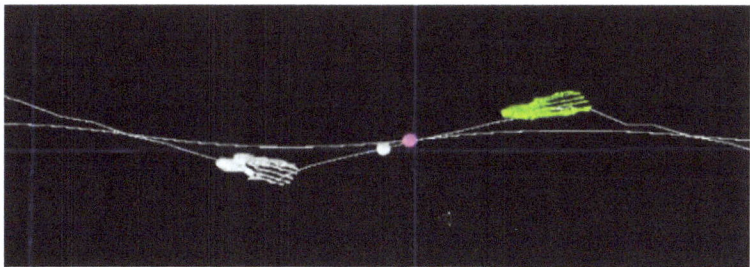

We want to observe here that the base of support must be placed appropriately to control the position of the COG. In this sense, to remain balanced while walking is to change the COP according to the position and velocity of the COG. It can be said that the base of support is properly arranged. In this way, walking is never a stable state. Instead, it would be more accurate to say that the unstable state is continuous.

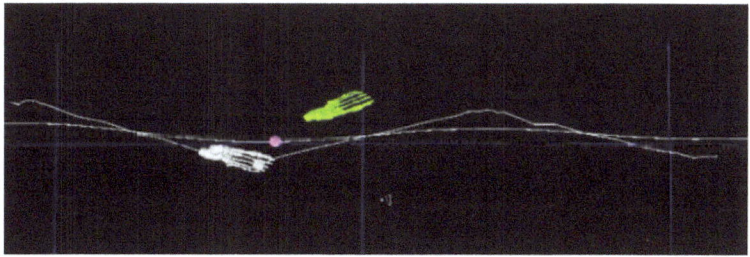

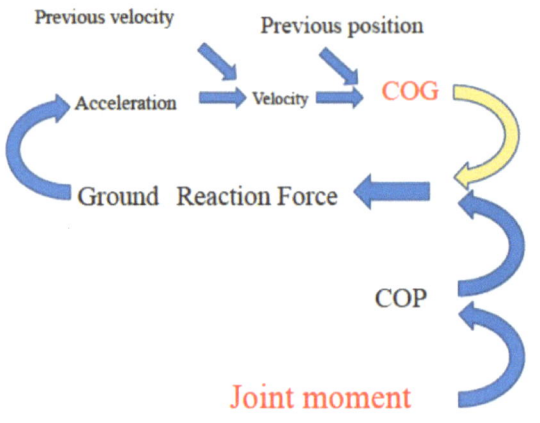

This figure resembles the Chapter 11 summary on gait initiation with more details. The joint moment changes the position of the COP and the horizontal (anteroposterior / mediolateral) component of the ground reaction force generated by the difference between the position of the COP and the position of the COG. The force causes acceleration of the COG, and the COG moves to determine its new position. At this time, the position of the COG is not directly determined by the force. It is the acceleration that is determined. This acceleration is added to the current velocity, and the new velocity is determined. The accumulation effect of this velocity finally determines the COG position. Therefore, control of muscle activity must be decided with all of these in mind. Walking is a much more complex movement than we can imagine.

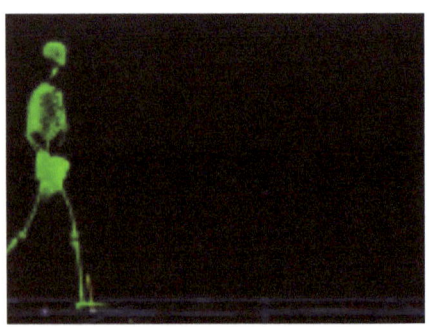
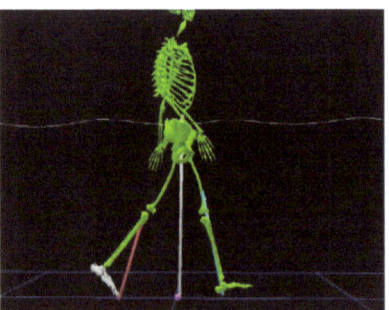

The Relationship between the Movement of COG and the GRF

Now that we know the mechanism by which the balance of the COG is maintained, let us look again at the relationship between the movement of the COG and the ground reaction force. The focus here is not the COP, but the ground reaction force itself. The COG moves forward while moving up and down smoothly. Let us start with the right foot touching the ground at the beginning of bilateral leg support. Focus on the ground reaction force. A backward ground reaction force is generated on the extended right foot and becomes greater at the same time that the direction is changed upward. On the other hand, the ground reaction force of the trailing left foot decreases gradually. Looking at the direction of both ground reaction forces, we can notice that the two vectors are not parallel. The forward ground reaction force is the propulsion force, and the backward ground reaction force is the deceleration force, so the front foot decelerates while the back foot propels. It seems like something strange, but when you think about it as a whole, the effects of propulsion and deceleration are just the same. This is why normal walking maintains an almost constant velocity. If the effect of propulsion is greater, we will accelerate more and more. This situation occurs during gait initiation. If deceleration is effective, the velocity will eventually become zero. This situation represents the end of the walking movement.

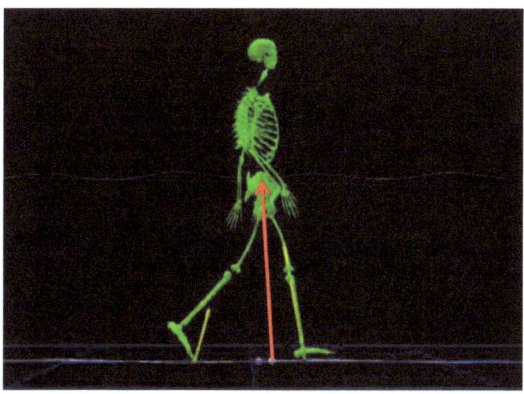

Let us focus on the combined ground reaction force of the left and right feet. First, look at the vertical component that corresponds to the height of the left and right ground reaction force vectors. The red arrow during the double-leg support period is quite long. In other words, the vertical component of the ground reaction force is larger (than gravitational force). During double-leg support, the COG sinks from a higher position, and reaches the lowest point, and again moves upward. This timing corresponds to the action of squatting down and using knee extension to stand back up. Recall that the ground reaction force is now greater than the gravitational force.

The COG rises during the single-leg support period. The ground reaction force at this time is smaller than the gravitational force. The COG reaches the highest point just above the support leg. Keep in mind that the upward movement is already decelerated before reaching the highest point. Otherwise, when reaching the highest point, the vertical velocity of the COG would not be zero. In this way, when the COG sinks and the descent changes to a rise, the ground reaction force becomes greater than the gravitational force. On the other hand, the ground reaction force becomes smaller than the gravitational force for a while after the mid-rise and past the highest point. It means that the height of the COG and the length of the ground reaction force are inversely related.

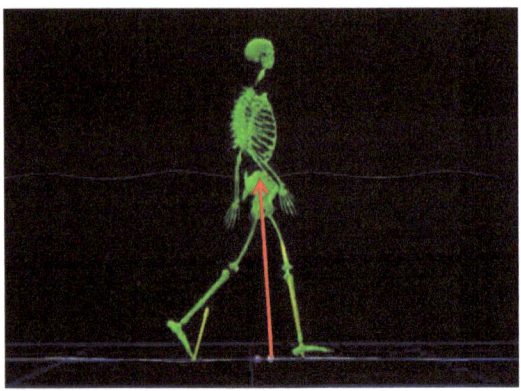

Now focus on the ground reaction force in the anteroposterior direction. The combined COP is located behind the COG for a while after the foot touches the floor, and you can see that the ground reaction force is leaning forward. In other words, the COG is accelerated forward at this time. When the COP is right below the COG (at the time of double support), the forward velocity becomes highest. After that, the COP overtakes the COG, the ground reaction force tilts backward, and the COG is decelerated. The forward velocity of the COG is the slowest when the COP moves directly under the COG (in the single-leg support period). Thus, the forward velocity of the COG is highest during the double support period and lowest during the single-leg support period.

Finally, pay attention to the ground reaction force in the medio-lateral direction. If you look at the frontal plane (from the posterior view), the ground reaction force vector is directed medially.

Therefore, the COG will meander inward, as seen from the support leg.

When the previously raised foot touches the floor, the ground reaction force of the foot turns outward, but immediately turns inward. Therefore, the combined ground reaction force gradually becomes inward in the single-leg support period of the extended foot. Then, the ground reaction force also turns inward (the reverse direction) **during the single support period of the opposite foot.** In other words, the COG always receives the inward force and does not move outside of the width of the left and right legs. With this mechanism, the COG moves forward while slightly meandering from side to side.

SUMMARY
While walking, the COG is never stable. In order to maintain stability, the human body relies on an excellent control mechanism.

CHAPTER 13

Functions to Smooth the Center of Gravity Movement During Gait

On completion of this chapter, you will be able:

1. To explain the function to smooth the movement of the center of gravity during walking
2. To explain the shock absorption mechanism during walking
3. To explain the relationship between the rocker function and the smooth movement of the center of gravity

This section describes the functions that enable a smooth center of gravity movement, a distinctive feature of healthy walking.

Functions to Smooth the Center of Gravity Movement during Walking

While walking, the center of gravity (COG) repeatedly moves up and down, where the COG is higher in the single-leg stance phase and lower in the double stance phase. The height of the COG when it is high is almost the same as when standing upright. During a single-leg stance, the COG position becomes slightly higher due to the rise in the COG of the swing leg side. The COG becomes slightly lower as **supporting leg** hip joint adduction increases. As a result, the position of the COG is almost the same as when standing upright.

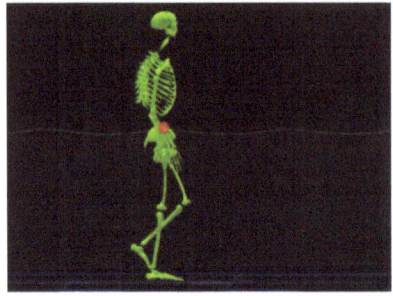

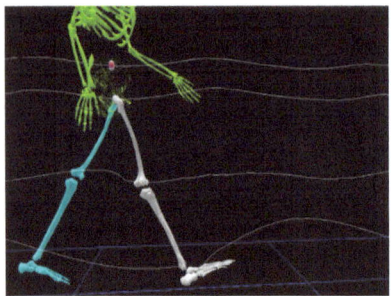

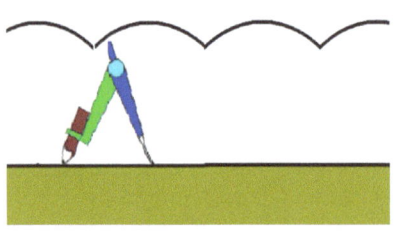

Compass walking

The COG position becomes lowest during the double support period. The difference in vertical height is about 3 cm, and the locus of the COG shows a smooth sine curve. The smoother the sine curve and the smaller the amplitude, the lower the energy consumption when walking. How does normal walking achieve a smooth and small-amplitude movement of the COG?

If a person's bipedal movement is like moving a compass as shown, the locus of the COG must draw a locus with a sharp valley. There are two ways to reduce the amplitude of this trajectory. One is to lower the height of the single-leg support period. Another is to increase the height during the double-leg support period. Considering the posture of the single-leg support period, it seems difficult to make it lower than the current position. Therefore, determining how to raise the COG during the double-leg support period is the key to reducing vertical movement.

In that sense, look at the posture of initial contact (IC). Initial contact is the timing of foot contact to the floor. The leading (front) leg strikes the floor with the heel. The trailing leg that remains behind stands on the toes. If you compare this posture with the posture where the soles of both legs are on the floor, you can notice that the COG is clearly higher. First, before the front foot touches the floor, decelerations occur with the ankle plantar flexor muscles of the back foot, and the heel is lifted to keep the COG high. This action corrects the trajectory so that the direction of the COG is not too downward.

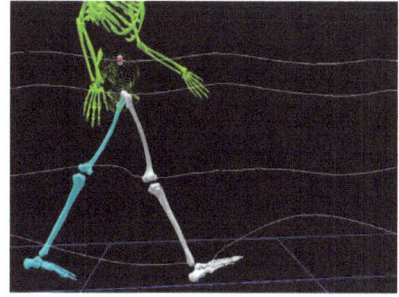

📝 For teachers

Please bring one student in front. Let him or her stand upright. Move the right leg in front and stop. This posture is just like a double support phase during walking.

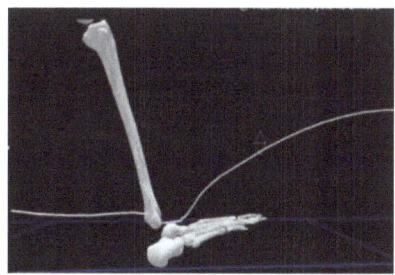

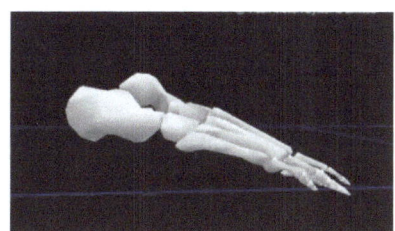

Let the student's back foot stand on the toes and the front foot on the ground with heel. At this time, remember the height of the head and compare the height to when the entire soles of both feet touch the floor.

Observing the front foot, it appears that landing with the heel allows the foot to rotate forward around the heel. The ankle can then move forward and downward.

What happens if you touch the toe instead of the heel? The foot will rotate backward with the toe as the center of rotation, and the ankle joint will move backward and downward.

Loading Response (LR) is the duration between the IC and the opposite foot's lift off from the floor. In the LR, the front foot heel comes in contact with the ground, the foot rotates around the heel, and the ankle turns forward and downward. This motion eliminates the need to correct the trajectory of the COG suddenly upward as in compass walking.

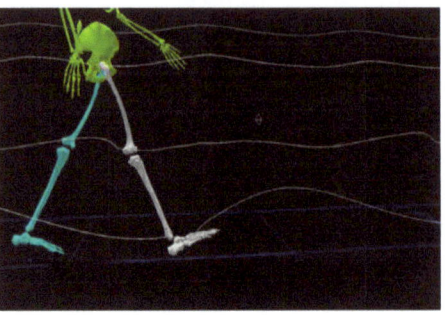

Center of gravity sinks after touchdown

During this period, the shank rises as much as the ankle joint goes down, and the knee can move horizontally to the floor. The knee joint flexes slightly, which causes the thigh to move horizontally at an almost constant angle relative to the floor. This motion allows the hip joint to move horizontally to the floor. The movement of the COG is almost the same as the movement of the hip joint, and the COG can move forward almost horizontally on the floor. Then, the knee will extend, and the entire lower limb will stand upright, so the COG will go upward.

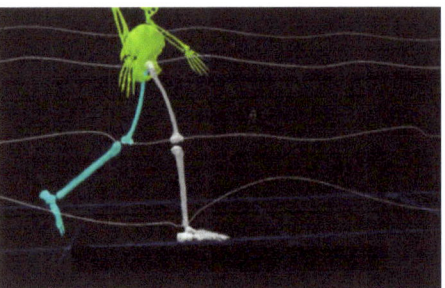

COG becomes higher

Midstance is the duration between the opposite foot's lift off and the observed foot's heel lift off the floor. In the second half of midstance (Mst), the entire lower limb rotates forward around the ankle

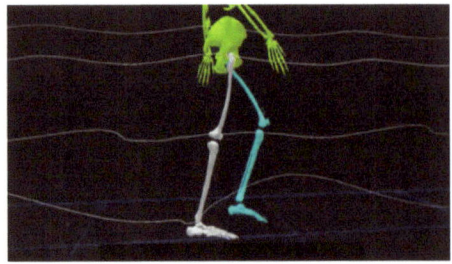

joint. The COG falls lower after the midstance. The right foot that was the front foot becomes the back foot, and the same situation is repeated. The joint movement described above makes the locus of the COG a smooth curve.

Shock Absorption Mechanism during Walking

Let us look at these series of movements from a different perspective. A big impact occurs when the front foot comes in contact with the ground. When the foot touches the ground, it is the same as the fall from a height of about 1 cm. Let's experience the shock at this time. Let us stand and raise the heel about 1 cm and feel the impact when dropping down. You can feel that the whole body is impacted. In human walking, this level of impact is applied to the grounded foot at every step, but we do not feel this impact. Why does this happen?

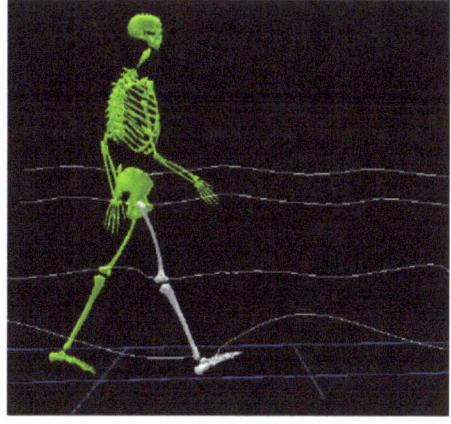

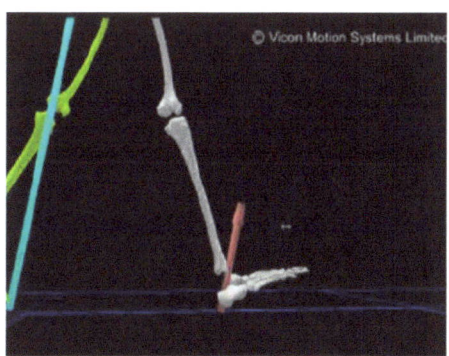

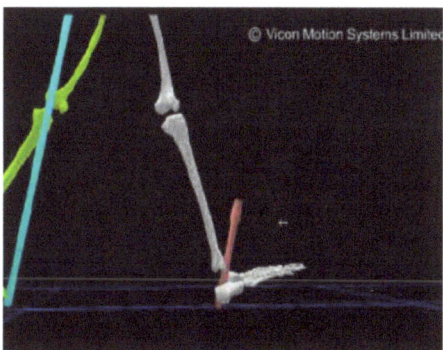

At initial contact during regular walking, the landing normally occurs at the heel. The heel has soft tissues of the skin, and there is cushioning from the shoes, so there is easily shock absorption. The toes are not structured to easily absorb shock because there is a period when the entire body must be supported by just one foot.

When landing on the heel, the ground reaction force rises from the heel and passes slightly behind the ankle. The ground reaction force tries to plantarflex the foot, but the ankle dorsiflexor muscles resist this by eccentric contraction. In other words, the eccentric contraction allows you to decelerate ankle plantar flexion. Thus, one of the purposes of the muscle's eccentric contraction is to absorb shock.

This figure shows the timing just slightly after the front foot touches the floor during loading response. At this time, the ground reaction force passes behind the knee and tries to flex the knee. The knee extension muscles are eccentrically contracted and decelerated to allow the knee to flex slowly. Again, shock can be absorbed by the eccentric contraction of the muscles.

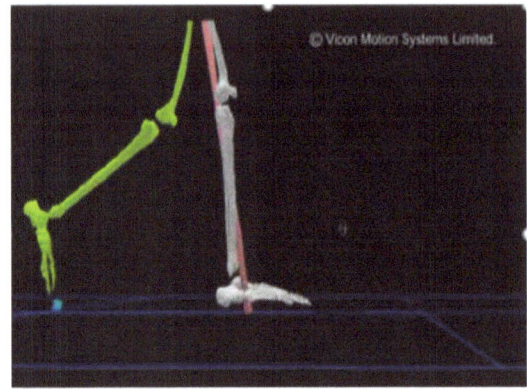

Interestingly, shock absorption begins before ground contact of the front foot. In the terminal swing (Tsw) of the front foot, the plantar flexors have an eccentric contraction in the ankle joint of the foot left behind. This plantar flexor action decelerates the body that has fallen forward. Without this deceleration, the burden on the front leg would be even greater.

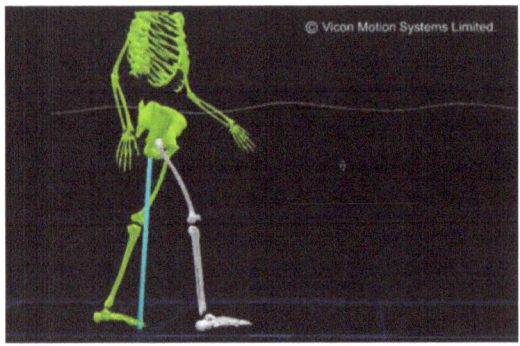

Rocker Functions and the Movement of COG

Heel rocker

Finally, let us look at these movements from the perspective of the rocker function. From the time of initial contact to loading response, the foot rotates forward around the heel. The OGIG (Observational Gait Instructor Group, U.S.A.) observed this function and expressed it in terms of heel rocker. A rocker is a chair that rotates the entire body forward and backward while the person sits on it. The heel rocker function plays an important role in absorbing the impact at ground contact and smoothing stance phase. With the heel rocker, the COG moves slightly forward and downward then becomes higher.

Fundamental Biomechanics

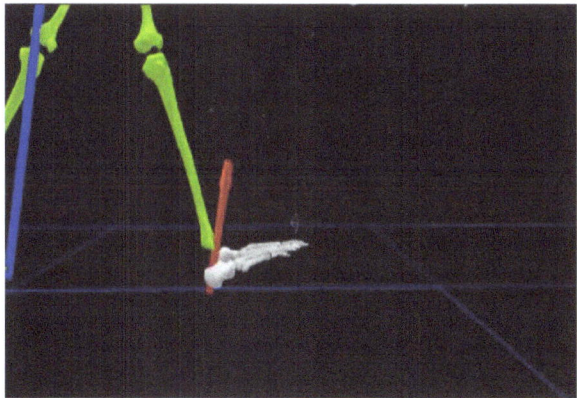

Ankle rocker

In midstance, when the foot is fully grounded to the floor, the ankle joint is now the center of rotation. This motion is an ankle rocker. The ankle rocker function occurs in an unstable single leg support period, and the ankle plantar flexor muscles apply an appropriate deceleration to the forward movement of the COG. It advances the COG smoothly. The COG during ankle rocker rises and then descends.

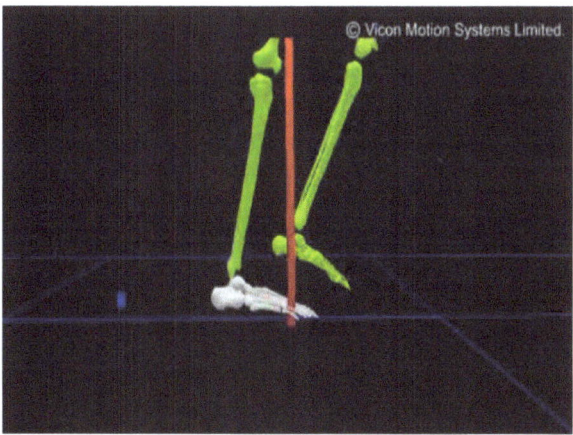

Forefoot rocker

When the load further moves to the forefoot, the heel floats and progresses into terminal stance (Tst). Terminal stance is the duration between the heel's lift off from the floor and the contact of the opposite foot to the floor. Tst has an important function for positioning the opposite foot. In Tst, the forefoot is the center of rotation. This motion is a forefoot rocker. The forefoot rocker continues from terminal stance to the pre-swing and plays a role in smoothly shifting the COG from the back foot to the front foot. The COG during the forefoot rocker moves forward while descending gradually.

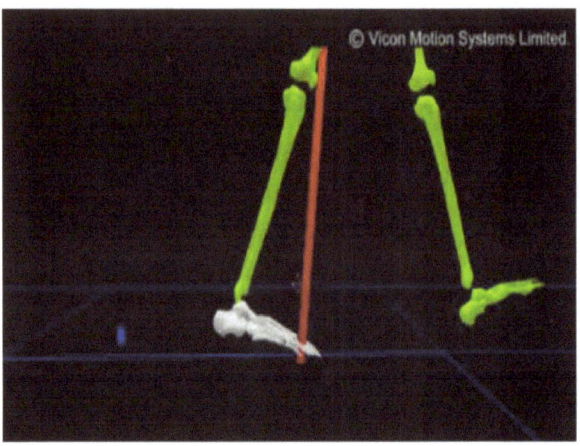

SUMMARY

The rocker function of normal walking is an excellent mechanism that smoothly rotates the body forward while moving the center of rotation gradually. This movement can only be completed with all three rockers, like a hop, step, and jump. Healthy people can easily carry the COG forward with less energy, properly negotiating the instability of walking as opposed to struggling with this instability. A proper knowledge of normal gait analysis can serve as a launchpad for learning about gait of physically challenged and older persons, which can be useful during rehabilitation.

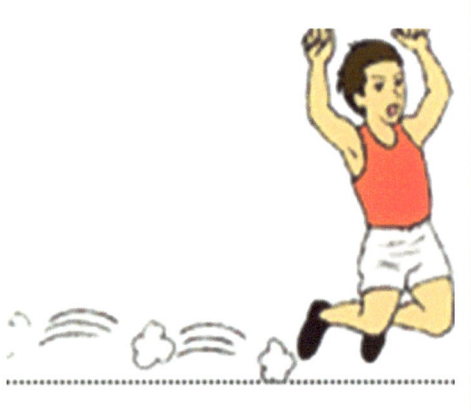

CHAPTER 14

Observational Gait Analysis OGIG method Observational Gait Instructor Group

On completion of this chapter, you will be able:

1. To explain OGIG gait terms
2. To explain the standard joint angle of healthy subjects in each gait cycle
3. To explain the three rocker functions

Here, students will learn how to observe normal gait using OGIG (Observational Gait Instructor Group) terminology. First, let us explain how to divide one gait cycle by OGIG terminology.

Observational Gait Analysis OGIG method Observational Gait Instructor Group

Gait cycle							
Classification by floor contact							
Stance				Swing			
Classification by function							
Transfer of the load		Single support		Swing of leg			
Initial Contact	Loading Response	Mid Stance	Terminal Stance	Pre Swing	Initial Swing	Mid Swing	Terminal Swing

This table shows one gait cycle.

One cycle is divided into stance phase and swing phase from the viewpoint of floor contact. From a functional point of view, the gait cycle is divided into load transfer, single support, and swing leg periods. The load transfer period is further divided into initial contact and loading response. The single support period is divided into midstance and terminal stance. The swing leg period is divided into the pre-swing (swing leg preparation period), initial swing, mid-swing, and terminal swing. OGIG defines eight terms for each gait cycle.

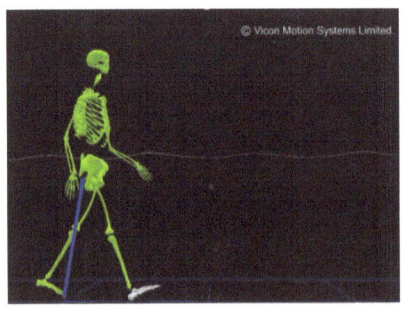

Initial Contact

First, for the sake of convenience, one gait cycle starts with the landing of one foot (for example, the right foot). The timing of ground contact by the foot of interest is called initial contact and is abbreviated as IC.

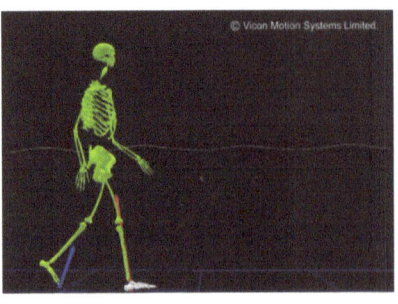

Loading Response

Since initial contact is the moment of touching the floor, it will end immediately.

The period from the right foot contact to the release of the left foot is called the loading response and abbreviated as LR.

Midstance

In the next period, the sole of the foot of interest (right foot) is on the ground. During this time, the opposite leg is moving forward away from the floor. Eventually, the heel of the right foot will float, and the period until heel float is called midstance and abbreviated as Mst.

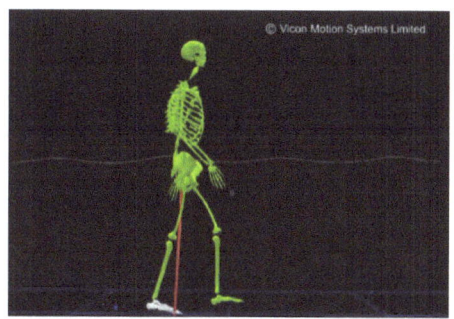

Terminal Stance

After the heel of the right foot floats, the initial contact of the left foot occurs. This period is called terminal stance and abbreviated as Tst.

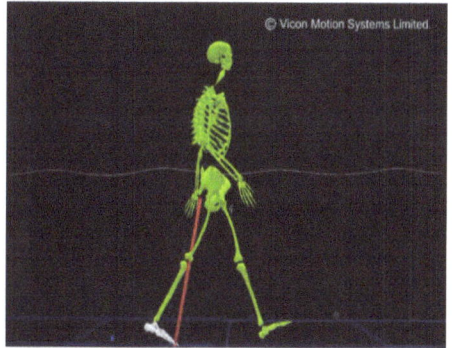

Pre-Swing

The period from the initial contact of the opposite foot (left foot) until when the right foot leaves the floor is called pre-swing, and the abbreviation is Psw. The target (right) foot is in contact with the floor, but from a functional point of view, it is classified as a preparation for swing phase. The pre-swing of the foot of interest is the loading response of the opposite foot.

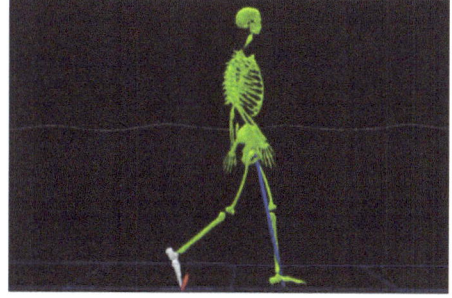

Initial Swing

The process from when the right foot leaves the floor and swings forward until it crosses the opposite foot is called the initial swing, and the abbreviation is Isw.

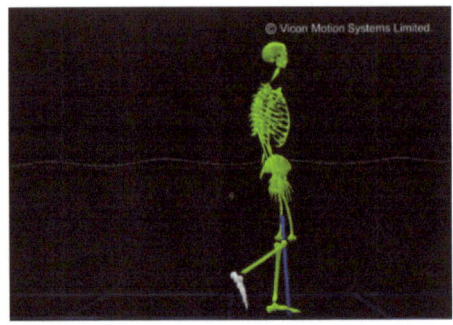

Midswing

The process until the shank of the swinging leg is vertical is called midswing and the abbreviation is Msw.

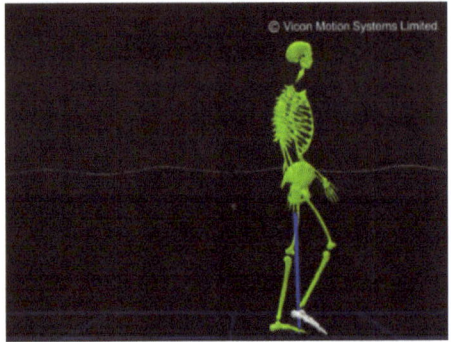

Terminal Swing

The process until the right foot makes initial contact again is called terminal swing and the abbreviation is Tsw. Thus, one gait cycle starts from the initial contact of the right foot to the initial contact of the right foot again. Naturally, one gait cycle starts from the initial contact of the left foot to the initial contact of the left foot again. Regardless of where you start, the time for one cycle is basically the same. "Basically" infers that a person is walking at the same rhythm every time.

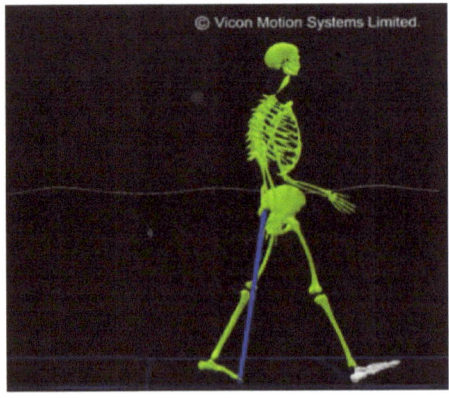

The time of one step is the time from the initial contact of the right foot to the initial contact of the left foot. The time of the next step is the time from initial contact of the left foot to the initial contact of the right foot. After all, it will be the same time whether you measure from the right or from the left foot.

Fundamental Biomechanics

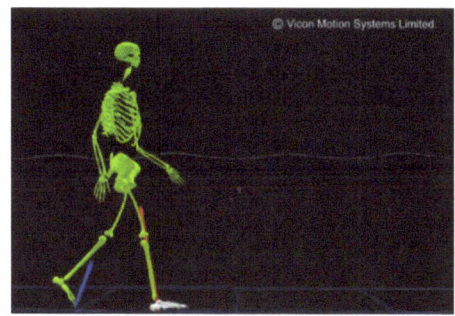

📋 For teachers
This is the end of the explanation of the gait cycle. Stop the computer graphic and playback from time to time to allow students to explain what each period represents.

Gait cycle							
Classification by floor contact							
Stance				Swing			
Classification by function							
Transfer of the load		Single support		Swing of leg			
Initial Contact	Loading Response	Mid Stance	Terminal Stance	Pre Swing	Initial Swing	Mid Swing	Terminal Swing

Let's revise the gait cycle again.

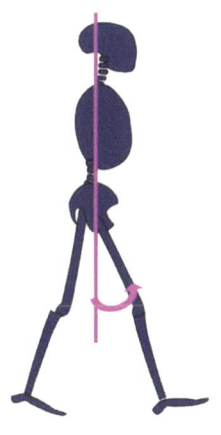

Normal Gait Analysis
After learning each phase of gait, let us learn about the average joint angle of a healthy person in each phase.

In this case, you should be careful about how to measure the angle of the hip joint. In OGIG gait observation, the angle of the hip joint is not based on the pelvis but the vertical line. The hip joint angle is expressed as how many degrees it flexes and what degree it extends with respect to the vertical line.

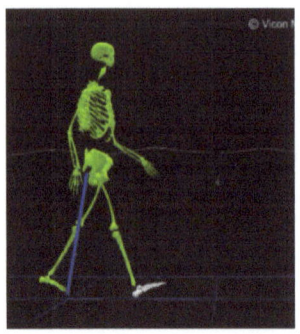

In initial contact, the pelvis is rotated 5° forward, the hip joint is flexed 20°, the knee joint is flexed 5°, and the ankle joint is 0°.

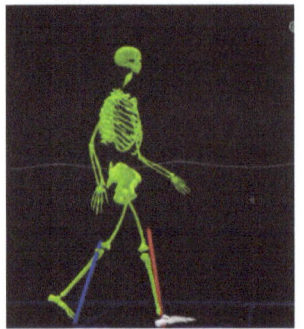

From here, the joint angle is expressed at the end of each phase.

At the end of the loading response, the knee joint is flexed 15°, and the ankle joint is plantarflexed 5°.

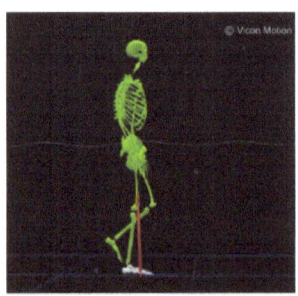

At the end of midstance, the hip joint is at 0° position, the knee joint is flexed 5°, and the ankle joint is dorsiflexed 5°.

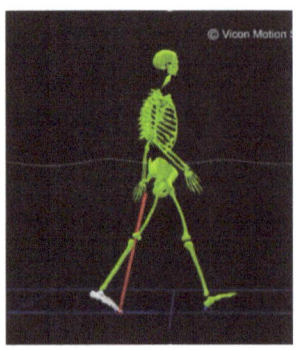

At the end of terminal stance, the pelvis is rotated 5° backward, the hip is extended 20°, the knee is flexed 5°, and the ankle is plantarflexed 10°.

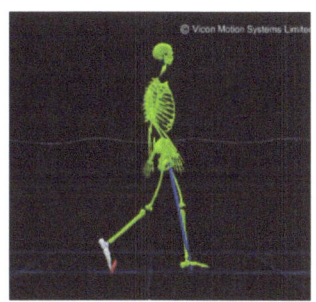

At the end of pre-swing, the hip joint is extended by 10°, the knee joint is flexed by 40°, and the ankle joint is plantarflexed by 15°.

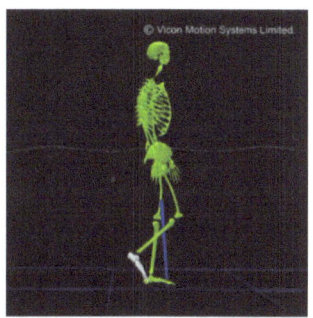

At the end of initial swing, the hip joint is flexed by 15°, the knee joint is flexed by 60°, and the ankle joint is plantarflexed by 5°.

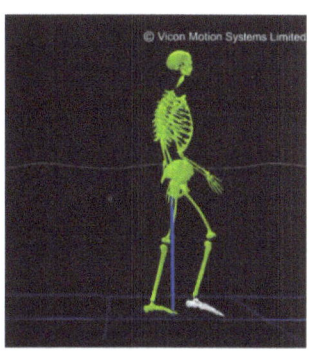

At the end of mid-swing, the hip joint is flexed by 25°, the knee joint is flexed by 25°, and the ankle joint is 0°.

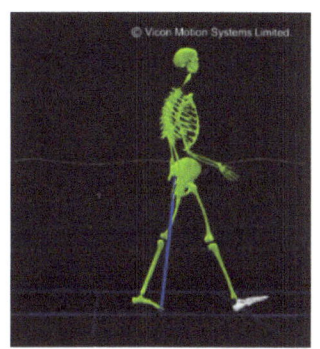

At the end of terminal swing, the pelvis is rotated 5° forward, the hip joint is flexed by 20°, the knee joint is flexed by 5°, and the ankle joint is 0°.

For teachers

Pause the computer graphic randomly and let the students answer the joint angle at each phase.

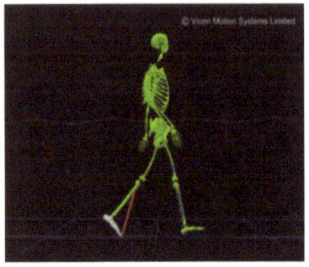

Rocker Functions Mechanism

Next, we will focus on where the axis of the foot and the body rotate during the stance phase of normal gait.

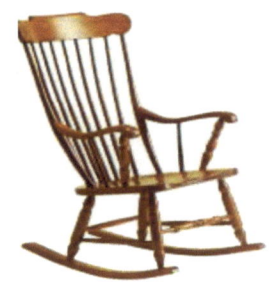

According to OGIG terminology, the body is moving like a rocking chair while walking. It is said that during the stance phase of healthy gait, rotation like a rocking chair occurs when the rotation axis moves. Such rotation is called a rocker function.

Let us take a look at the three rockers.

First, at initial contact, let us check whether the heel touches the floor first. Healthy people always touch the floor with the heel. The foot rotates forward, with the heel as the center of rotation, during the loading response. This function is called a heel rocker. Inappropriate rotation with the heel is expressed as incomplete heel rocker or insufficient heel rocker.

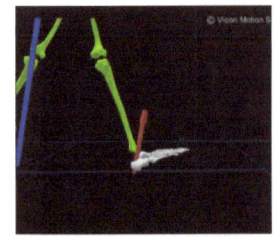

In the following midstance, the sole touches the floor, and the body rotates forward around the ankle joint. This function is called an ankle rocker. When the rotation at the ankle joint is inappropriate, it is expressed as an incomplete ankle rocker or insufficient ankle rocker.

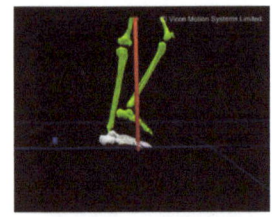

In terminal stance, the heel floats, and the foot rotates forward with the forefoot as the center of rotation. This function is called a forefoot rocker. If

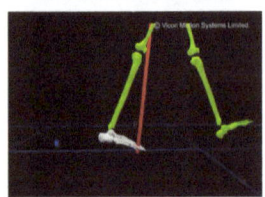

the rotation of the forefoot is inappropriate, it is expressed as incomplete forefoot rocker or insufficient forefoot rocker.

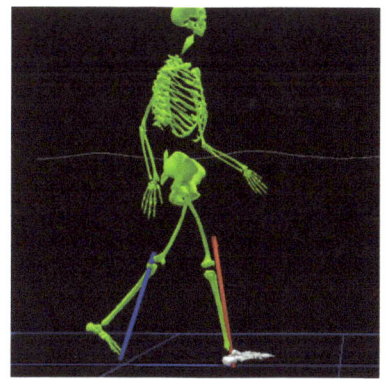

Let us look at muscle activity during gait while drawing the rocker function in mind. When considering joint moments that represent muscle activity, it is important to look at the relationship between ground reaction forces and joint positions. First, let us take a look at the ground reaction force.

Let us focus on the movement of the ground reaction force in the sagittal plane. The force is almost upright in the single-leg support period and has a large inclination in the double-leg support period. The ground reaction force of the rear leg tilts forward, and the ground reaction force of the front leg tilts backward. The rear leg kicks the floor backward, then receives the force of the accelerator and pushes the COG forward. At the same time, the front leg decelerates and prevents a sudden forward movement. In normal gait, the accelerator and decelerator are repeated at each step.

Let us take a look at the relationship between the ground reaction force and the joints, with the inclination of the ground reaction force in mind. Roughly speaking, it can be said that the ground reaction force is clinging to the lower limbs while changing the inclination. Therefore, the ground reaction force and joint position are not greatly separated throughout one gait cycle. This indicates that there is no significant muscle activity during gait of healthy individuals, especially around the knee and hip joints.

Let us consider muscle activity around the ankle joint from the viewpoint of the rocker function. Please watch the computer graphic focusing on the relationship

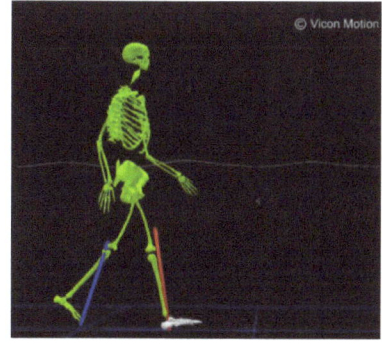

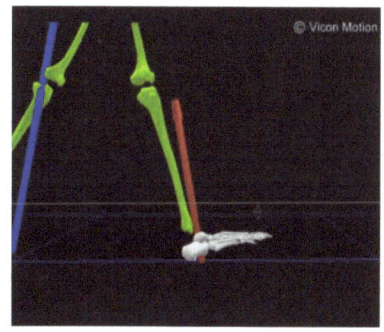

between the ankle joint and ground reaction force. In the heel rocker, the ground reaction force passes slightly behind the ankle, and you can see that the dorsiflexor is active. At this time, the ankle joint is plantarflexed, causing the dorsiflexor to undergo eccentric contraction. Eccentric contraction of the dorsiflexor reduces the impact when touching the ground and smoothly rotates the entire body forward.

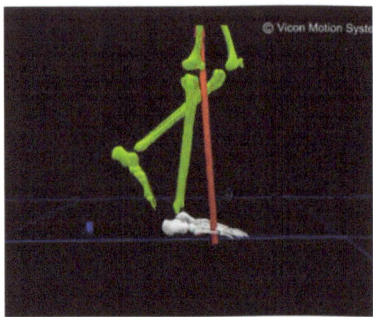

In the ankle rocker, the ground reaction force passes through the front of the ankle joint, and you can see that the plantar flexor muscles are active. At this time, the ankle joint is dorsiflexed, so the forward movement of the COG is decelerated by the eccentric contraction of the plantar flexor muscle.

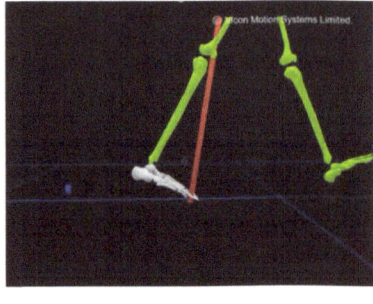

In the forefoot rocker, the ground reaction force passes largely in front of the ankle joint. At this time, there is an increase in the activity of the plantar flexor muscles leading to a load on the toes that allows a larger stride, while the opposite foot moves forward. The forefoot rocker plantar flexor is the most active during the gait cycle.

SUMMARY
At the end of this chapter, you should:

- Understand the gait cycle.
- Learn the standard values of joint angles in each phase.
- Understand the rocker function mechanism.

List of quoted figures

Manga Biomechanics I
(Biomechanics expressed by Comic), in Japanese
Nanko_Do, Tokyo, Japan 1994

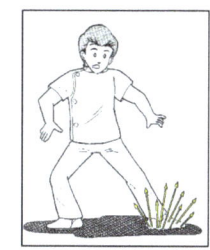

Human Anatomy for CG creators
, in Japanese
Born Digital, Inc., Tokyo, Japan

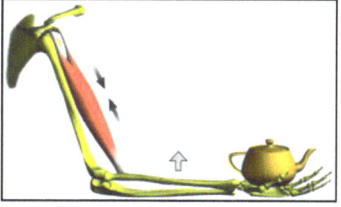

Chapter 14 is based on the concept of OGIG method.

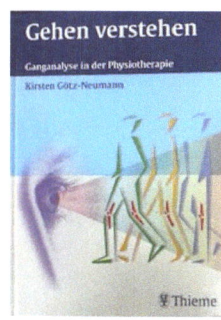 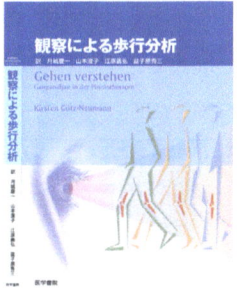

www.gehen-verstehen.de

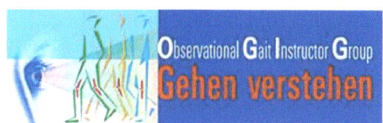

www.ingramcontent.com/pod-product-compliance
Lightning Source LLC
Chambersburg PA
CBHW041947240526
45473CB00036B/2411